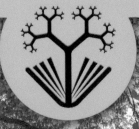

MORE THAN
STRESS

Understanding Anxiety Disorders

CHERRY PEDRICK, RN / BRUCE M. HYMAN, PhD
TABITHA MORIARTY

TWENTY-FIRST CENTURY BOOKS / MINNEAPOLIS

Thank you to Kerri Pedrick for her assistance and advice. *More Than Stress* is dedicated to the millions of people who struggle daily with anxiety disorders, the families whose lives are deeply affected by anxiety disorders in their loved ones, and the doctors, researchers, and scientists who dedicate their lives to helping patients with anxiety disorders and finding more effective treatments.

Twenty-First Century Books™
An imprint of Lerner Publishing Group, Inc.
241 First Avenue North
Minneapolis, MN 55401 USA

For reading levels and more information, look up this title at www.lernerbooks.com.

Diagrams on pages 8, 12, 21, 36 by Laura K. Westlund.

Main body text set in Conduit ITC Std.
Typeface provided by International Typeface Corp.

Library of Congress Cataloging-in-Publication Data

Names: Pedrick, Cherry, author. | Hyman, Bruce M., author.
Title: More than stress : understanding anxiety disorders / Cherry Pedrick, R.N., Bruce M. Hyman, Ph.D.
Description: Minneapolis : Twenty-First Century Books, [2023] | Series: Healthy living library | Includes bibliographical references and index. | Audience: Ages 11–18 | Audience: Grades 10–12 | Summary: "Many teens struggle with anxiety disorders, the symptoms of which include elevated stress hormone levels, depression, and heart problems. The prevalence of anxiety disorders among teens today makes this a timely, informative, and helpful book for readers. Readers will learn about the causes, symptoms, and diagnosis of anxiety disorders as well as coping strategies and treatments. Resources for identifying, managing, and treating anxiety disorders are provided in the text"— Provided by publisher.
Identifiers: LCCN 2021040627 (print) | LCCN 2021040628 (ebook) | ISBN 9781541588936 (library binding) | ISBN 9781728419114 (ebook)
Subjects: LCSH: Obsessive-compulsive disorder—Juvenile literature.
Classification: LCC RC533 .P43 2023 (print) | LCC RC533 (ebook) | DDC 616.85/227—dc23

LC record available at https://lccn.loc.gov/2021040627
LC ebook record available at https://lccn.loc.gov/2021040628

Manufactured in the United States of America
1-47456-48021-2/25/2022

CONTENTS

LIVING WITH ANXIETY

When someone uses the term *anxiety* or shares that they are feeling anxious, what do they mean? *Anxiety* is a word often used to describe a specific worry. This type of anxiety tends to focus on a specific event in the near future. For example, someone may say that they are feeling anxious about their upcoming performance in a play or asking their crush out on a date. Generally, when the word *anxiety* is used this way, the person speaking is referring to this common feeling of nervous anticipation.

Anxiety can also mean something different. When someone talks about experiencing a clinical anxiety disorder, they are talking about a specific category of mental health disorders that causes a lot of distress and can affect many facets of everyday life. In this book, we will discuss some of the many recognized clinical anxiety disorders and the effects that they have on people's daily lives. Many people struggle with clinical anxiety disorders every day, and the different types of disorders and their symptoms can look different on different people. It's important to talk about anxiety disorders to raise awareness and decrease stigma around them. People experience anxiety disorders for many reasons, and with treatment many enjoy life with few or no symptoms.

So what is clinical anxiety? Some people describe this anxiety as an intense fear. Fear is a normal, healthy part of the human experience. It is an appropriate response to threats, challenges, and potential loss. Fear encourages you to study harder for tests, reminds you to get college applications in on time, and makes you take reasonable safety precautions. Worry stemming from such fears is helpful and helps us succeed, argues Luana Marques, an associate professor of psychiatry at Harvard Medical School and president of the Anxiety and Depression Association of America. "Worry is a way for your brain to handle problems in order to keep you safe," she explains. "It's only when we get stuck thinking about a problem that worry stops being functional." When fear is out of proportion to the threats at hand and causes excessive worry about unlikely future events, the result is anxiety. Many people experience anxiety from time to time, especially when they are under stress from work, school, or relationship troubles. When anxiety persists and interferes with daily life, a person may be diagnosed with an anxiety disorder.

Fear vs. Anxiety

Fear is a response to a well-defined danger, a specific object, or a particular situation. Think of it as the brain's natural alarm system that goes off when there is a present threat. The level of fear one experiences is in proportion to the actual threat. Common fears include illness, job loss, family separation, physical harm, poverty, and death. Anxiety is an excessive, out-of-proportion response to a hypothetical, future-oriented danger. Someone experiencing anxiety may not be able to describe the actual threat. Often there might be just a sense of overwhelming panic that something bad will happen. Other people experiencing anxiety may be able to pinpoint a specific circumstance or event they fear. As the event draws near, or as they think about it often, they may experience even more severe anxiety. The event does not have to be something occurring in the near future. For example, a nine-year-old may experience a racing heart and intense fear when they think about whether they will pass their driver's test, even though their driver's test will not occur for many years. Someone else may feel anxiety at the thought that they and their loved ones will someday die of old age, even though that event may be years away.

Anxiety affects people on four levels. There can be many physical symptoms, including rapid heart rate, stomach discomfort (butterflies), trembling, nausea, muscle tightness, sweating, vomiting, diarrhea, and shortness of breath. Mental symptoms include uneasiness, worry, intrusive thoughts, confusion, poor concentration, and a sense of helplessness. Emotionally, anxiety might look like feelings of panic, embarrassment, or rejection. Anxiety may also manifest in behaviors, such as avoiding particular objects, places, or situations. As with obsessive-compulsive disorder (OCD), someone may perform unnecessary rituals. Recovery often involves treatment of the physical, mental, emotional, and behavioral aspects of the symptoms. Some people may experience anxiety on only one of the four levels or more intensely on one of the levels. When this occurs, recovery and treatment will focus on alleviating the symptoms that are causing distress.

Anxiety starts with the body's natural fear response to perceived threats. Our senses of sight, hearing, touch, taste, and smell pick up signs of danger in our environment. The brain evaluates the information and begins to prepare the body for fight or flight. The same process prepared our ancestors to run from an attacking grizzly bear or to stay and fight the bear to the end. The threats and dangers of modern society involve threats to our self-worth, our self-esteem, our sense of personal security, our health, and our safety. When someone is experiencing an anxiety disorder, the brain responds to all these threats the way it would respond to an attacking grizzly bear.

Certain areas of the brain analyze incoming information and control emotions. When the brain perceives a threat, an activating chemical called adrenaline is released into the bloodstream. Adrenaline causes the heart to race, blood pressure to rise, and breathing to quicken. When this response helps you flee a burning building, the response is healthy and protective. A healthy fear response furthers your survival and helps you do your best. When the fear response is overactivated and becomes anxiety, it can harm you instead of protect you.

It's useful to think of anxiety as an excessive activation of the body's natural fear response. Anxiety is what occurs when the brain's fight-or-flight mechanism becomes mistakenly associated with objects, places, people, situations, or ideas that we don't normally think of as very threatening. For example, if someone was swimming in the ocean and saw a black fin rise out of the water a few feet from them, and the lifeguard hollered, "Shark in the water!" their heart would start racing. They would gasp for air and start thrashing their arms to get as far away from the shark as quickly as possible. Someone with anxiety may have that same heart-pumping, "Got to

FIGHT-OR-FLIGHT RESPONSE

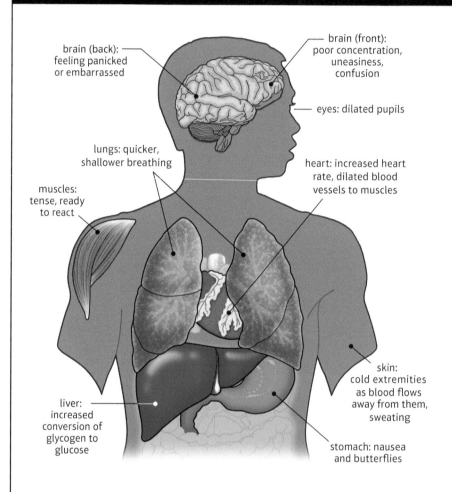

brain (back): feeling panicked or embarrassed

brain (front): poor concentration, uneasiness, confusion

eyes: dilated pupils

lungs: quicker, shallower breathing

muscles: tense, ready to react

heart: increased heart rate, dilated blood vessels to muscles

skin: cold extremities as blood flows away from them, sweating

liver: increased conversion of glycogen to glucose

stomach: nausea and butterflies

Humans evolved the fight-or-flight response as a survival mechanism to react quickly to life-threatening situations. In stressful situations, stress hormones trigger a series of physiological reactions.

get away right now!" reaction not only in the presence of a real shark but while watching a movie about sharks, looking at a picture of sharks, seeing any fish that resembles a shark, or just being within a few feet of the ocean.

Reactions like these are what behavioral scientists sometimes refer to as the brain's "false alarms." Despite knowing that no threat is currently present, the brain triggers a fight-or-flight reaction anyway, causing great distress. These false alarms become learned and ingrained by the repeated association of the fearful object or situation (such as bees, zoos, heights, door locks, and blood) with the brain's fight-or-flight response. They are the basis of anxiety disorders.

What Causes Anxiety Disorders?

According to the National Institute of Mental Health, 19.1 percent of US adults will have experienced an anxiety disorder in the past year, and 31.1 percent of US adults will experience an anxiety disorder in their lifetimes. People with anxiety need to know that they are not alone. Science is providing more and more solid clues in the search for greater understanding of the causes of anxiety disorders. Our best knowledge to date indicates that anxiety disorders are caused by a multitude of factors—biological, genetic, psychological, and environmental. Each factor contributes in varying degrees to a person's unique vulnerability to developing an anxiety disorder.

Research suggests that some people genetically inherit extra-sensitive fight-or-flight warning systems from their parents. They seem to be born alert, nervous, or worried. Their bodies overrespond to harmless stimuli as if they were dangers. Studies of the genetics of identical twins have demonstrated how anxiety disorders tend to run in families. Identical twins have almost exactly the same genetic makeup. Several studies have shown that when an identical twin has an anxiety disorder, the other twin is more likely to have an anxiety disorder. This is less likely with fraternal twins, which hints that our genetic makeup plays a role in the development of anxiety disorders.

Other factors enter the picture soon after birth. Environment, upbringing, and stress can combine to make it more or less likely that someone will develop an anxiety disorder.

Besides genetics and environment, biological and physical factors can influence the development of an anxiety disorder. Anxiety may result from neurochemical imbalances in the brain with

LIFE EVENTS AND ANXIETY DISORDERS

Researchers in Baltimore studied about 150 children to understand whether certain life events contribute to the development of anxiety disorders. The scientists interviewed first graders and their parents, and then interviewed them again six years later, when the children were in seventh grade.

The study identified six events that might predispose children to developing anxiety disorders. These six events are loss-death, loss-separation, social adversity, negative family environment, academic difficulties, and peer rejection. Examples of these include experiencing the death of a sibling, grandparent, or pet (loss-death); parental divorce (loss-separation); eviction (social adversity); having a parent with a substance use disorder (negative family environment); having difficulties in school or undiagnosed learning disabilities (academic difficulties); or experiencing bullying or feelings no known cause. Doctors can prescribe drugs that help to correct this neurochemical imbalance. Certain medical conditions may also cause symptoms of anxiety and panic. These include some heart conditions, some lung conditions, problems with the balancing system in the inner ear, hormone irregularities, allergies to food additives, low blood sugar, and some vitamin deficiencies. Treating these conditions often eases the accompanying anxiety. Some people may experience anxiety as a side effect of drug or alcohol use, especially when using stimulants such as caffeine or nicotine. Withdrawal from drugs and alcohol can also result in feelings of anxiety and panic.

of social isolation (peer rejection). Of these six categories, researchers found that children who experienced loss-death, academic difficulties, or a negative family environment experienced more anxiety symptoms.

In an interview with CNN, therapist Claire Bidwell Smith explains how experiencing one or more of these life events, especially death, can trigger anxiety symptoms. "When some big change comes seemingly out of nowhere and disrupts life, we realize we're not safe, things aren't certain, we're not in control. . . . That feeds anxiety."

Many people experience several of these events and do not develop an anxiety disorder. Others may develop an anxiety disorder after experiencing one of these events. The development of an anxiety disorder is dependent on many factors, not just life experiences. For example, two siblings might have the exact same upbringing with the same challenging experiences, and one could develop an anxiety disorder while the other does not.

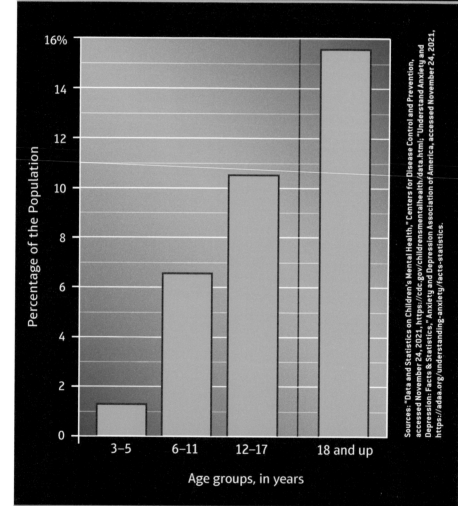

PERCENTAGE OF POPULATION WITH AN ANXIETY DISORDER BY AGE GROUP

Percentage of the Population

16%

14

12

10

8

6

4

2

0

3–5   6–11   12–17   18 and up

Age groups, in years

Sources: "Data and Statistics on Children's Mental Health," Centers for Disease Control and Prevention, accessed November 24, 2021, https://cdc.gov/childrensmentalhealth/data.html; "Understand Anxiety and Depression: Facts & Statistics," Anxiety and Depression Association of America, accessed November 24, 2021, https://adaa.org/understanding-anxiety/facts-statistics.

While anxiety disorders are most common in adults, a significant number of children and teens also develop anxiety disorders.

Some people can find evidence of anxiety disorders within many branches of their family tree, perhaps pointing to a genetic influence. Others can identify traumas such as severe childhood neglect or abuse as triggers in the development of their anxiety disorder. Still others may experience anxiety as a side effect of a medical illness. Because the causes of anxiety disorders are complex, so are the treatments. Treatments aim to rebalance brain chemistry, change harmful beliefs and self-defeating behaviors, retrain the way people interpret interactions with others, and reduce stress through positive lifestyle changes. An individualized treatment plan can make living with an anxiety disorder much more manageable.

CHAPTER ONE

PANIC AND FEAR

S ome anxiety disorders have specific triggers. A person with one of these disorders experiences anxiety symptoms when faced with a particular situation or object, and they will often avoid being put into circumstances where they may encounter that situation or object. This chapter will look at the symptoms and root causes of these specific anxiety disorders.

Panic Disorder

Panic disorder is a fairly common condition that affects about 4.7 percent of the US population. It consists of two major components. The first is the panic attack, an initial frightening experience of brief but very intense fear that occurs unexpectedly. The second component is an ongoing preoccupation with the fear of having

HOW DOCTORS DIAGNOSE

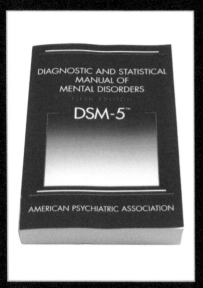

This book bases the criteria for diagnosing each anxiety disorder on the fifth edition of the *Diagnostic and Statistical Manual of Mental Disorders*, or *DSM–5*. It was written by a large group of leading experts in the field of psychiatry and mental health and is the manual for officially diagnosing mental health disorders. This edition was published in 2013.

The *DSM–5* updated requirements for diagnosing specific disorders, reclassified certain disorders, and introduced new diagnoses that were not included in the previous edition.

another panic attack in the future. Most people who experience panic disorder have their first panic attack in their late teens or early twenties. Much more rarely, a person will have their first attack before the age of sixteen or after fifty. A person can be considered to have panic disorder if they have any of the following symptoms:

- recurrent, unexpected panic attacks
- persistent worry, for a month or more, about having future attacks

- worry, for a month or more, about what the attacks may mean (such as thinking "I'm losing control" or "I've had a heart attack")
- a change in behavior due to the attacks (such as avoiding certain places, driving long distances, or other situations for fear of having another panic attack) that lasts for a month or more
- panic attacks that are not due to organic factors (such as taking in too much caffeine) or a general medical condition (such as an overactive thyroid or low blood sugar)
- panic attacks that are not due to another mental disorder (such as substance use disorder)

Panic attacks are sudden waves of severe anxiety that begin abruptly. The symptoms usually last only a few minutes, although they can return in waves for a couple of hours. What does a panic attack feel like? At least four of the following symptoms are present in full-blown panic attacks. (If only two or three are present, it's called a limited-symptom attack.)

- racing or pounding heart (palpitations)
- sweating
- trembling or shaking
- shortness of breath (dyspnea)
- feeling of tightness in the throat or choking
- chest pain or discomfort
- nausea or abdominal distress
- feeling dizzy, unsteady, or faint
- feeling unreal or detached

- numbness or tingling sensations (paresthesia)
- chills or hot flashes
- fear of dying
- fear of insanity or losing control

Having a panic attack can feel scary and isolating. Someone who is having a panic attack doesn't always understand what is happening until after the attack is over, especially if they have not

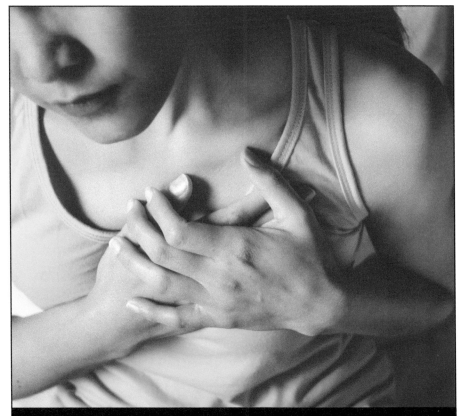

During a panic attack, the body's fight-or-flight response kicks in. Physical symptoms are usually severe and disruptive.

had many in the past. Panic attacks can occur anywhere, and in addition to panic attack symptoms, the person may be anxious about how their attack looks to the people around them. Someone who experiences panic attacks may withdraw from the people in their lives because they don't want to be seen as weak. But having panic attacks does not make someone weak. Panic attacks can happen to anyone.

Agoraphobia

Panic attacks can be terrifying. The fear of having another panic attack can be even worse. A person who has panic attacks often can become intensely focused on avoiding the physical sensations—such as rapid heartbeat, sweating, shortness of breath, and muscle tension—that accompany their panic attacks. These sensations are associated with specific situations where escape is difficult, where help is either unavailable, or where getting help will attract the attention of others.

The pattern of avoiding places and situations that feel unsafe is called agoraphobia. The word *agoraphobia* comes from Greek words meaning "fear of the marketplace." For a person with agoraphobia, the anticipation of public (marketplace) humiliation and loss of control is as terrifying as the panic sensations themselves. Agoraphobia affects around 1 percent of the population. Many people are diagnosed with both panic disorder and agoraphobia.

Someone with agoraphobia may feel fear in enclosed areas, crowded places, open spaces, and while home alone. Areas that can cause fear include elevators, tunnels, bridges, stores, open fields, theaters, restaurants, hair salons, and public transportation vehicles. Often fear responses are triggered by being a certain distance from home or outside city limits. People with agoraphobia also try to avoid situations that have a high probability of triggering panic sensations. A person who fears the sensation of shortness of breath, for example, may consistently avoid climbing a flight of stairs, doing strenuous exercise, or being in a stuffy, crowded room.

Many people with agoraphobia only feel safe going outside with a "safe person." This person is often a spouse, parent, or close friend. They are aware of the fears and avoidance patterns of the agoraphobic person and are seen as someone who can provide safety during a panic attack. In addition, some people with agoraphobia feel they must have particular objects such as

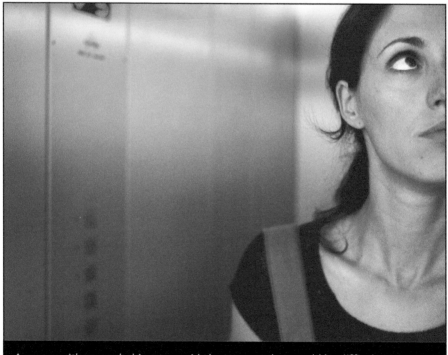

A person with agoraphobia may avoid elevators, as they would be difficult or impossible to escape in the case of a panic attack.

tranquilizers, cell phones, or bottles of water while out in areas they consider unsafe. The mere thought of going out without one of these safety objects can cause anxiety to spike.

People with agoraphobia often describe their fears as if they have a fear of specific places, such as shopping malls or elevators. Usually their fear is actually of the bodily sensations and distressing thoughts that they associate with specific places and situations. For this reason, panic disorder and agoraphobia (as well as the other anxiety disorders) have often been described as the "fear of fear."

What Causes Panic Disorder and Agoraphobia?

Why do some people develop panic disorder and agoraphobia? Research points to a genetic predisposition toward being excessively anxious and apprehensive. These individuals may have extra-sensitive fight-or-flight systems. The parts of the brain that activate the process—which include the amygdala, the anterior cingulate cortex, and the locus coeruleus—get set off without any apparent threat, like a car alarm that goes off when no one is near. The brain sends adrenaline racing through the body, causing the heart to beat faster and breathing to speed up.

A person's experience and history are important aspects when assessing vulnerability to panic disorder. They determine in part whether an individual will interpret a particular physical sensation as dangerous or harmless. The most important factor may be the environment in which a person was raised. Research studies have shown that early experiences with uncontrollable events such as family illness, death, and other traumas may increase vulnerability to developing anxiety disorders. For example, parents who focus

THE HUMAN BRAIN AND PROCESSING FEAR

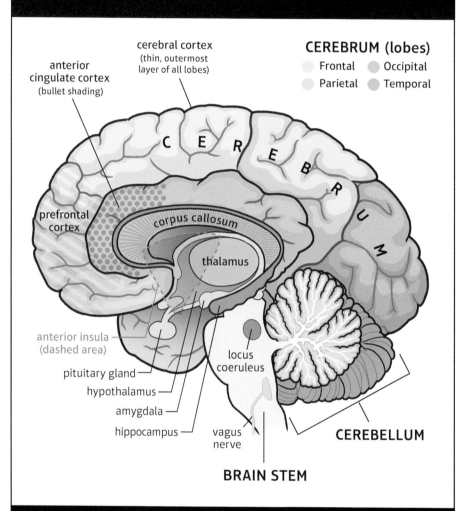

cerebral cortex
(thin, outermost
layer of all lobes)

anterior
cingulate cortex
(bullet shading)

CEREBRUM (lobes)
- Frontal
- Occipital
- Parietal
- Temporal

C E R E B R U M

prefrontal
cortex

corpus callosum

thalamus

anterior insula
(dashed area)

pituitary gland

hypothalamus

amygdala

hippocampus

locus
coeruleus

vagus
nerve

CEREBELLUM

BRAIN STEM

The amygdala detects stimuli that we should pay attention to in our environment. The anterior cingulate cortex takes information from the amygdala and determines the appropriate bodily response. The locus coeruleus then adjusts the amount of adrenaline in the bloodstream.

intensely on the fear and prevention of illness in their children may predispose them to overfocus on the dangers of bodily sensations as adults.

Most people report a period of significant life stress preceding their first panic attack. Stressful life events such as illness, death of a loved one, divorce, a job change, a move, or a personal loss can set the process of emotional hyperarousal in motion. This can lead to a panic attack in someone who is predisposed to panic attacks or anxiety. While many people respond with curiosity or annoyance to a sudden rapid pulse, this predisposed person may have a panic attack. After experiencing one or even a few panic attacks, someone may develop a fear of having another panic attack.

Panic disorder might not be triggered by any one significant life event. Sometimes a combination of smaller stressors may build up over time and cause a panic disorder to develop.

Social Phobia

Social phobia, also known as social anxiety disorder, affects 12.1 percent of the US population. The disorder often starts during adolescence, when social relationships take on immense importance. People with this disorder experience severe anxiety in social situations. They fear the scrutiny of others, which might make them feel embarrassed or humiliated. They may also fear that others will not understand what they are experiencing and make incorrect judgments or assumptions about them.

This anxiety is far worse than the nervous butterflies most people feel in new social situations such as a first date, a party, or a job interview. Mild to moderate nervousness can help motivate people to make the best impression they can on others and is not considered unhealthy. For someone with social phobia, the fear is intense enough to interfere significantly with a person's normal routine, school or work functioning, social activities, or relationships. The person also feels great distress about having anxiety.

A person with social phobia may dread or avoid social situations such as parties, meetings, and job interviews. Activities that can cause discomfort include talking to strangers or authority figures such as teachers, dating, public speaking, performing, participating

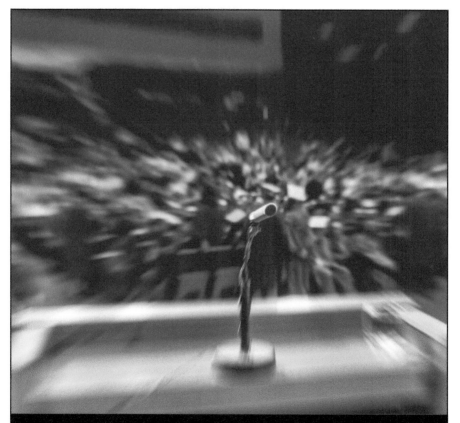

Someone with stage fright may experience trembling in the hands and legs, rapid heart rate, sweaty hands, dry mouth, or other symptoms.

in sports, eating or drinking in front of other people, using public restrooms, and writing in front of other people. Reactions to social situations can vary from stomach pains, inner anxiety, muscle tension, and dry mouth to stuttering, sweating, and full-blown panic attacks.

Some people feel anxious only in specific situations. Fear of public speaking is the most common form of social phobia. This type of social phobia is also called stage fright, especially when it is a fear of musical, theatrical, or other artistic performance. When a person has anxiety around a number of social situations, it is sometimes called generalized social anxiety disorder.

A variety of factors can contribute to developing this disorder. People who develop the disorder appear to be born with a genetic predisposition to developing social phobia. This type of anxiety disorder tends to run in families. But just having a genetic predisposition for it does not mean a person will develop it. Environmental factors can also play a role. For example, some patients report that their parents were critical and overprotective. A child in this environment may be shy and timid. Studies have shown that children who are shy and timid are more likely to develop social phobia, although these traits on their own are not necessarily causes for concern.

Some studies examine the differences in the brains of people with and without social phobia. One study was conducted at Duke University in North Carolina in 1994. A team of researchers used magnetic resonance imaging (MRI) scans to compare the brains of people with social phobia and the brains of people without the disorder. They found that a structure in the middle part of the brain, called the putamen, shrank in size more rapidly with age in the patients with social phobia. The putamen produces a neurotransmitter, or chemical messenger, called dopamine. Dopamine affects feelings of pleasure in the brain. A shrinking putamen could produce less dopamine than the body needs. Other research also indicates imbalances in the way social phobia patients' brains handle the neurotransmitters dopamine and serotonin. Antidepressants, which boost levels of dopamine and serotonin in the brain, can be used to treat these chemical imbalances in patients with anxiety disorders. The relationship between anxiety and depression, along with specific treatments, will be discussed in more detail later in this book.

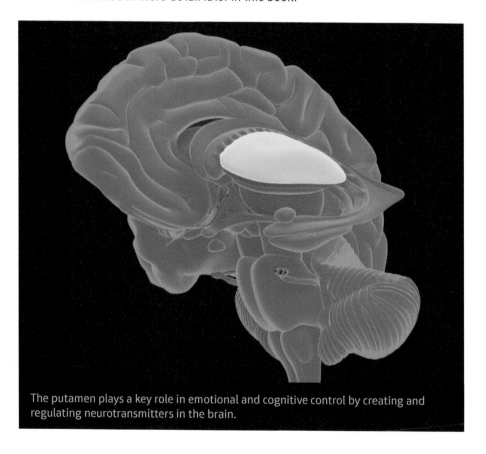

The putamen plays a key role in emotional and cognitive control by creating and regulating neurotransmitters in the brain.

SOCIAL MEDIA ANXIETY DISORDER

With the rise of social media, society has become more interconnected than ever. Individual use of social media varies widely, with some people using it every day and others avoiding it completely. For most, social media is a communication tool or a source of entertainment. But some develop an unhealthy patten of use.

Social media anxiety disorder is a diagnosis that, while not yet added to the *DSM–5*, is becoming increasingly common. This anxiety disorder shares many similarities with social phobia, but social media is the main trigger for the disorder. Someone experiencing social media anxiety disorder may obsessively check social media to see what people are doing without them. They might compare themselves and their real lives to the curated and edited images they see online. A person with this disorder may link their self-worth to the number of followers they have or the number of likes they receive on a post. They might think that their social standing in real life depends on these online relationships. They may also experience feelings of anxiety if they are not tagged correctly in photos or if they receive comments that they perceive to be unflattering or critical. People with this anxiety disorder often spend more than eight hours a day on social media. Side effects can include body image issues, low self-esteem, and worsening isolation from real life.

In December 2021, US surgeon general Vivek Murthy issued a report warning that young people are facing devastating mental health effects in part due to the media they are consuming. "Young people are bombarded with messages through the media and popular culture that erode their sense of self-worth—telling them they are not good-looking enough, popular enough, smart enough, or rich enough," he wrote in the report.

Social media may help people to connect with one another, especially people who live long distances apart or are unable to see one another due to other circumstances such as illness. Not all use of social media has negative consequences. Just as with other anxiety disorders, social media anxiety disorder becomes a problem when it has a significant and negative impact on a person's life or when it begins to cause them severe distress.

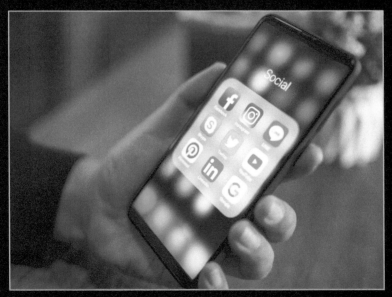

Researchers have found that people who have social media anxiety disorder are more likely to suffer from depression and attention-deficit/hyperactivity disorder.

Specific Phobias

People with specific phobias have an excessive or unreasonable fear of one particular type of object or situation and actively avoid it. When they do encounter it, they feel intense fear and anxiety, even panic. Typical specific phobias include fears of snakes, spiders, dogs, cats, flying, heights, water, blood, needles, and dental procedures. Almost anything can be the object of a phobia. Here is a small sample of the vast range of possible specific phobias:

- agrizoophobia—fear of wild animals
- arachnophobia—fear of spiders
- claustrophobia—fear of confined spaces
- coprophobia—fear of feces
- electrophobia—fear of electricity
- emetophobia—fear of vomiting
- equinophobia—fear of horses
- hydrophobophobia—fear of rabies
- ichthyophobia—fear of fish
- lockiophobia—fear of childbirth
- triskaidekaphobia—fear of the number thirteen

About 8.7 percent of the US population experiences specific phobias. As with other anxiety disorders, the tendency to develop phobias appears to run in families. Genetic factors can predispose a person to develop phobias. Some fears may be learned from parents. A young child can develop a phobia by observing a parent with a similar fear. Phobias can also develop after a traumatic event, such as a disaster, an accident, or an illness. A specific phobia may not cause a problem in the person's life until it becomes impossible for the person to continue to avoid the feared situation or object. For example, the fear of heights could overwhelm a person who gets a job in an office on the twenty-second floor of a building.

For those who suffer from anxiety, fear, and panic, help and hope are available. Thanks to increased scientific research over the past several decades, many medical doctors and therapists know a great deal about how to treat anxiety disorders and how to help people handle stress, anxiety, and fear. Additionally, the push to normalize and destigmatize mental health disorders has helped people feel more comfortable seeking help for all mental health disorders, including anxiety. Many college campuses, for instance, provide free mental health services for students. As more people become aware of the effects and prevalence of anxiety, the medical field will likely continue to find more effective treatments to help people recover from and manage anxiety disorders.

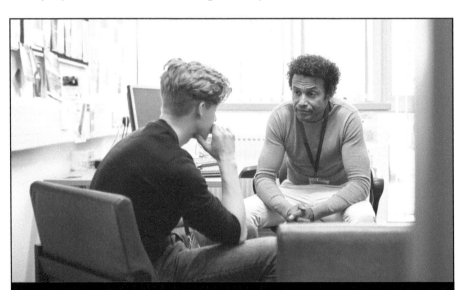

A 2012 study found that approximately 73 percent of students had experienced a mental health crisis while in college. Providing easy access to academic accommodations, clinical services, and crisis services means these students can receive the help they need to thrive on campus.

CHAPTER TWO

RITUALS, TRAUMA, AND WORRY

The anxiety disorders in the previous chapter are triggered by very specific situations. Other types of anxiety disorders have a broader scope. These disorders may affect an individual on every level of functioning or may intensify without warning. For example, someone suffering from agoraphobia may only experience symptoms when in crowded places, while someone suffering from OCD may experience anxiety symptoms in multiple aspects of daily life—at home, at work, at school, while eating meals, or when spending time with friends. Someone experiencing generalized anxiety disorder (GAD) may suffer from constant feelings of anxiety with few or no identifiable triggers. This is different from someone experiencing social phobia, where the anxiety is specific to social situations. Someone experiencing post-traumatic stress disorder (PTSD), for example, may experience signs and symptoms of trauma when triggered by specific incidents but also at times that seem random. These conditions can generate even more anxiety, as the person does not know when or where the next attack will happen.

This chapter will provide an overview of these types of anxiety disorders. While this section will cover common symptoms and causes, people with these anxiety disorders may experience only some of these symptoms or may have different symptoms than the ones mentioned here.

Obsessive-Compulsive Disorder

In the United States, about 2.3 percent of the population has OCD. Most people begin to experience symptoms before the age of thirty, in childhood or adolescence, but can also have a later onset. People with OCD experience persistent thoughts, impulses, ideas, or images they cannot ignore. The ideas and images cause such intense anxiety and distress that people with OCD feel they must do something to get relief.

Compulsions, or rituals, develop in an effort to relieve the distress and anxiety brought on by obsessions. These compulsions are repetitive behaviors that can include checking, cleaning, repeating actions, and arranging objects in a particular order. They can also be repetitive mental acts such as praying, counting, repeating words silently, and going over events in one's mind. Some people may also experience symptoms such as skin-picking, hair-pulling, or nail-biting.

People with checking compulsions have irrational fears of terrible things happening to themselves or others because of things they do or don't do. They may check door locks or household

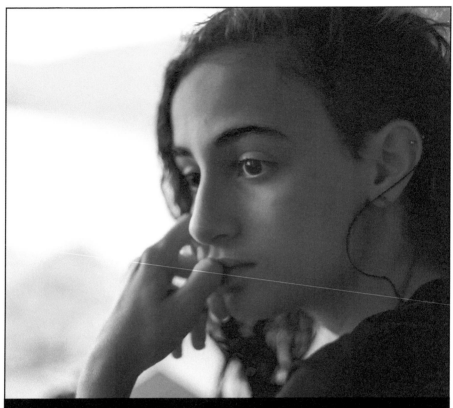

Nail-biting is one example of a repetitive behavior that can become a compulsion.

appliances or check their homework and test questions repeatedly. Those with washing and cleaning compulsions may wash their hands, shower, or clean their surroundings to ease excessive fears about contamination by germs, dirt, or foreign substances. Others arrange certain items in precise ways. Books or papers might be kept in a particular order. Some people repeat behaviors in a specific order or insist on a certain kind of precision, such as shoelaces or socks being perfectly even. A few people with OCD have a compulsion to collect or hoard items.

Compulsions are often linked to a vague goal of preventing or avoiding death, illness, or another dreaded event. There may or may not be a relationship between the compulsion and the dreaded event. A person might check the arrangement of books on a shelf as a response to an obsessive thought about harm coming to a loved one, for example. In this instance, there is no direct relation between the obsession and the compulsion. OCD manifests in a variety of ways. Checking, washing, and cleaning compulsions are the most common, but there are many other types of compulsions.

Some people with OCD have mental compulsions rather than behavioral compulsions. They have unwanted, intrusive, horrific thoughts and images of causing danger or harm to others or themselves. They never act upon these thoughts. Instead, to ease their distress, many people with OCD purposefully engage in repetitive thoughts such as counting or repeating certain words. They may also mentally review distressing situations as a way of preparing themselves in case these situations occur again. Some people with obsessive thoughts that center on religious and moral issues—called scrupulosity—may compulsively pray or repeat religious scripture to ease their anxiety. The compulsive thoughts and mental reviews help at first but soon prove inadequate to relieve the anxiety. Cycles of obsessive and compulsive thoughts take up increasing amounts of time—almost every waking hour in many cases.

Whatever the compulsions—checking, washing, ordering, or praying—performing them once won't be enough. The list of things to be checked or washed grows, because relief is only temporary. The anxiety and distress return, and more compulsions are needed. Of course, most people have had some obsessive thoughts. And hasn't everyone checked and rechecked a test or double-checked to

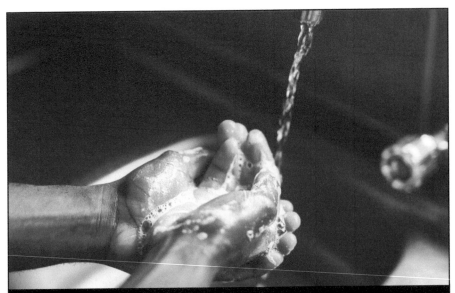

Certain compulsions, such as handwashing, come with their own health concerns. Excessive handwashing can result in itchy, dry, or blistering skin. Bacteria can enter through cracks in dry skin and create sores.

make sure the door was locked? Only when obsessive-compulsive behavior significantly interferes with daily living—with functioning at home, school, or work—or when it causes a great deal of distress to the person is the condition likely to be diagnosed as OCD.

OCD tends to run in families, so there appears to be a genetic predisposition for the condition. An imbalance in the mood-stabilizing neurotransmitter serotonin plays a role in OCD. Brain imaging studies have shown abnormalities in several parts of the brains of people with OCD, including the orbitofrontal cortex, thalamus, basal ganglia, caudate nucleus, and cingulate gyrus.

Occasionally, OCD can develop suddenly in children as a reaction to strep throat. Experts believe the body forms antibodies against the streptococci bacteria, and these antibodies then attack

TRICHOTILLOMANIA

Trichotillomania is a disorder that causes people to compulsively pull out their hair. It is a disorder closely related to OCD.

Symptoms of trichotillomania include the following:

- repeatedly pulling hair out, typically from the scalp, eyebrows, or eyelashes but sometimes from other body areas
- noticeable hair loss, such as shortened hair or thinned or bald areas on the scalp or sparse or missing eyelashes or eyebrows
- repeatedly trying to stop pulling hair or trying to do it less often without success
- significant distress or problems related to pulling hair at work, at school, or in social situations

A person with trichotillomania may begin to pick at their hair with a conscious intention of pulling it. In other cases, it may be an automatic behavior when the person is doing something else such as watching TV or studying. The consequences of trichotillomania can vary, but they can include severe hair loss, damage to the scalp and eyeballs, the formation of a trichobezoar (a large hair ball in the stomach as a result of eating the hairs), and social isolation. Treatments for trichotillomania mainly use therapy to help patients manage. Currently no medications have been approved for trichotillomania, although some doctors may prescribe an antidepressant as a part of treatment.

THE HUMAN BRAIN AND OCD

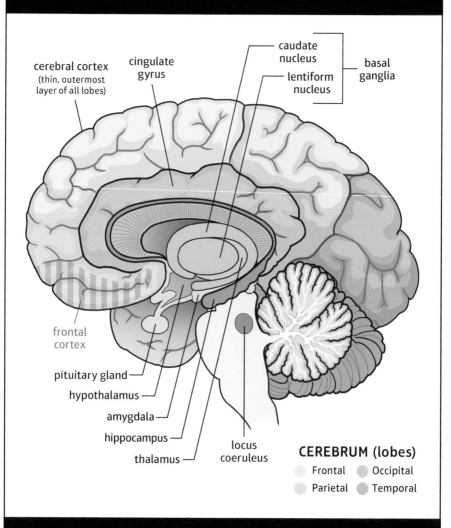

cerebral cortex
(thin, outermost
layer of all lobes)

cingulate gyrus

caudate nucleus

lentiform nucleus

basal ganglia

frontal cortex

pituitary gland

hypothalamus

amygdala

hippocampus

thalamus

locus coeruleus

CEREBRUM (lobes)
- Frontal
- Parietal
- Occipital
- Temporal

Studies suggest that abnormalities in the orbitofrontal cortex, thalamus, basal ganglia, caudate nucleus, and cingulate gyrus may be factors in the development of OCD.

certain structures within the brain. This leads to OCD symptoms or worsening of existing OCD symptoms. Symptoms can be treated quickly with traditional antibiotic medications that kill off the strep bacteria.

Particular traumatic experiences can also bring on OCD symptoms. Some people who develop OCD later in life have experienced stressful childhoods or a singular stressful or traumatic event. This event might be the sudden death of a loved one, homelessness, or a serious car accident. OCD can also occur after a traumatic brain injury. Someone may suffer the injury in a motor vehicle accident, when falling and hitting their head, or even from getting a concussion while playing sports.

Post-Traumatic Stress Disorder

The symptoms of PTSD have been described in psychiatric journals since World War I (1914–1918). Soldiers coming back from the war were said to have shell shock, soldier's heart, or war neurosis. They had anxiety, nightmares, and flashbacks for weeks, months, or years after coming back from fighting in the war. Psychiatrists later saw the similarities between the symptoms soldiers experienced and those of people who had experienced other devastating traumatic events such as accidents and natural disasters. This was eventually recognized as a specific psychiatric condition that develops after a person experiences severe trauma. PTSD was first established as a diagnosis in 1980.

Traumatic events such as sexual, physical, and emotional abuse; rape; assault; and witnessing disasters or death can lead to PTSD. People may also develop PTSD after events such as a motor vehicle accident or the unexpected death of a loved one. Different

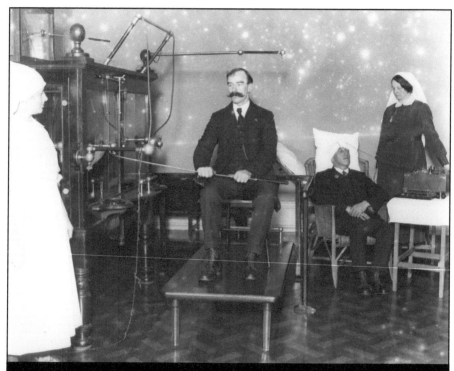

Nurses at the Sir William Turner's Hospital in England used experimental medical treatments to treat shell-shocked patients during World War I.

people's bodies process events differently. Two people may experience the same event, and one may develop PTSD while the other does not.

The symptoms of PTSD usually occur immediately after a trauma but occasionally surface years later, when a person is under further stress. For a person to be diagnosed with PTSD according to the *DSM–5*, they must have experienced, witnessed, or been confronted with an event that involved actual or threatened death or serious injury to themselves or others. Symptoms need to be present for at least one month, and they must cause significant distress or impairment. (If symptoms last for less than a month, the condition is classified as acute stress disorder.) Symptoms include

- persistent reexperiencing of a traumatic event in one or more of the following ways:
    - » recurrent and intrusive distressing recollections
    - » recurrent distressing dreams about the event
    - » acting or feeling as if the traumatic event were happening again
    - » intense psychological distress at exposure to things that resemble or symbolize an aspect of the event
    - » physical stress responses to cues that resemble or symbolize an aspect of the event

- avoidance and emotional numbness, as indicated by three or more of the following:
    - » avoiding thoughts, feelings, or conversations associated with the trauma
    - » avoiding activities, places, or people that trigger recollections of the trauma
    - » inability to recall an important aspect of the trauma
    - » markedly diminished interest or participation in significant activities
    - » feeling detached or estranged from others
    - » inability to have loving feelings
    - » having trouble imagining or planning for the future (such as expecting not to have a career, a family, or a long life span)

- symptoms of increased restlessness as indicated by two or more of the following:
  - » difficulty falling or staying asleep
  - » irritability or outbursts of anger
  - » difficulty concentrating
  - » hypervigilance
  - » exaggerated startle response

PTSD affects 3.5 percent of Americans. People with PTSD are also more likely to experience depression, panic disorder, GAD, social phobia, substance use disorder, or suicidal tendencies.

Many people experience horrendous traumatic events and don't develop PTSD. Many factors impact one's vulnerability to PTSD symptoms. Genetic makeup, certain childhood events, previous traumas, lack of social support, and limited coping skills can all contribute to the development of PTSD.

Generalized Anxiety Disorder

About 5.7 percent of Americans have GAD. The hallmark of GAD is worry—frequent, uncontrollable worry about negative events that either won't happen soon or have little chance of happening. People with GAD feel anxious and worry excessively on more days than not. For a person to be diagnosed with GAD, the anxiety and worry must last at least six months, and the person must worry about a number of events and activities, not just a few. In addition to anxiety and worry, people with GAD can feel restless, keyed up, on edge, fatigued, or irritable. They can also have difficulty concentrating, muscle tension, and sleep disturbances. To meet the criteria for a diagnosis of GAD, the anxiety and worry must cause significant distress or impairment and cannot be caused by a medical condition, substance use, or any other mental disorder. Everybody worries, but there is a difference between normal worry and the worry that people with GAD experience.

VETERANS AND PTSD

Military veterans are at increased risk of developing PTSD compared to the general population. While on active duty, veterans may have gone on missions where they experienced horrible or life-threatening situations. In addition to trauma personally experienced in combat situations, veterans may be exposed to other forms of trauma. A military doctor, for example, may experience cumulative trauma after treating numerous combat wounds.

Soldiers may also experience trauma in the form of sexual harassment or assault during their military service. Nearly one in four women veterans report being sexually assaulted while in the military; 55 percent of women and 38 percent of men reported being sexually harassed.

According to the US Department of Veterans Affairs,

- an estimated 30 percent of Vietnam War (1954–1975) veterans have had PTSD in their lifetime.
- approximately 12 percent of Gulf War (1991) veterans have PTSD in a given year.
- between 11 and 20 percent of veterans who served in Iraq and Afghanistan during Operations Iraqi Freedom and Enduring Freedom (2001–2014) have PTSD in a given year.

NORMAL WORRY	GAD WORRY
Focused on only a few future threats	Focused on many diverse future threats that have little or no realistic chance of happening
Helps a person prepare for coping with a future threat. It promotes healthy problem solving to deal with the threat.	Involves little effective problem solving and may interfere with problem solving
In proportion to the real threat being faced	Out of proportion to the threat being faced
Rarely incapacitating	Incapacitating

Generalized anxiety disorder tends to be persistent and chronic. Only 43.2 percent of people experiencing GAD are receiving treatment. Up to 90 percent of people with the disorder have another psychiatric disorder, most commonly clinical depression. Many also have physical symptoms that stem from chronic anxiety, such as headaches, irritable bowel syndrome, and stomach distress. They may visit their doctor much more than the average person without GAD does and may receive other diagnoses if their doctor does not correctly recognize their symptoms.

GAD appears to run in families. Twin studies indicate at least part of the cause is genetic, but apparently, environment also plays a major role. Family stressors such as divorce or excessive parental expectations contribute to the development of GAD, especially in adolescents. Stressful or traumatic events, such as a death in the family or a bad car accident, can be factors too.

ANXIETY AND LIFE STRESSORS

Life stressors can cause a person to develop an anxiety disorder as an attempt to cope with the problem. Life stressors can include the following:

- parental divorce or separation
- moving
- starting at a new school or university
- starting a new job
- death of a loved one
- searching for a college
- stress from school
- being diagnosed with an illness or having someone close be diagnosed with an illness
- financial stress or instability

Not all stressors may seem significant to outsiders, and that's OK. What matters is how the stressor affects the person with the disorder. Someone struggling with an anxiety disorder should never feel ashamed of the things they worry about or how they cope with specific stressors. The most important thing is to get help.

Biological factors also impact the likelihood of developing GAD. People with GAD frequently have an imbalance of neurotransmitters that help regulate mood. Medications that affect the absorption of these neurotransmitters are useful in treating GAD.

In addition to medication options, learning new ways to manage stress and handle stress-provoking thoughts are important to long-term treatment of GAD. Psychotherapies like cognitive behavioral therapy (CBT) can help individuals frame anxious thoughts and behaviors differently. Techniques such as breath work, or controlled breathing, can help people concentrate on their breath or body movement rather than on potential threats. Specific treatments and therapies will be discussed in depth in the next chapter.

CHAPTER THREE

TREATMENT OPTIONS

Anxiety disorders affect people on physical, mental, emotional, and behavioral levels. People with untreated anxiety disorders are at risk for the disorders worsening over time. They are also at risk for developing other anxiety disorders, depression, and substance use disorder. For these reasons, it's important to start treatment as early as possible.

The first step is a diagnosis by a qualified mental health professional, preferably a psychiatrist or a psychologist who specializes in treatment of anxiety disorders. The doctor typically reviews the patient's medical and psychiatric history and gathers information from the patient about their experiences with anxiety. The therapist then comes up with a treatment plan to address the patient's needs. This treatment may include psychotherapy, medication, a combination of both, or some other treatment.

How does a person find a qualified mental health professional? Most people begin by making an appointment with their family doctor, a school counselor, or a mental health clinic. Any trusted health provider in your community can direct you to a qualified mental health professional with a background, experience, and success in treating anxiety disorders. National organizations such as the Anxiety and Depression Association of America and the Association for Behavioral and Cognitive Therapies provide the names of doctors and therapists who list treating anxiety disorders as one of their specialties or interests. The organizations don't always track the treatment practices of these professionals, however. Checking a doctor's profile on their practice's website can reveal more about how they approach their work. It can also indicate whether they have experience in other areas relevant to the patient, such as trauma or abuse, family issues, or LGBTQIA+ issues. Patients may have to meet with a few different professionals before deciding on one who is a good fit.

You can check that a clinician's license is current by calling your state government's licensing board for that clinician's profession (such as medicine, psychology, or social work). Then you can find information about any disciplinary action taken against them. If any, you might consider going to a different clinician.

If medication is part of the treatment plan, the patient may need a psychiatrist. Psychiatrists are medical doctors who can prescribe medication. But not all psychiatrists are trained to provide psychotherapy, which can be very helpful in treating anxiety disorders. Some psychiatrists have sought this training, and many partner with psychologists or clinical social workers who provide psychotherapy such as CBT. If not, the psychiatrist should be willing to make a referral to someone who can.

THERAPY IS NOT ONE-SIZE-FITS-ALL

When people think of therapy, they often think of the pop culture trope of a therapist sitting in a huge armchair taking notes while the patient lies on a couch, looking up at the ceiling and talking about their childhood. While some therapist-patient relationships do function this way, there are many different types of therapy. Here are some:

- family-centered therapy
- group therapy
- cognitive behavioral therapy
- movement therapy
- art or music therapy
- equestrian therapy
- eye movement desensitization therapy

Perhaps even more important than the type of therapy is the therapist. Studies have shown that whether a patient is practicing CBT or traditional psychotherapy, their condition improved more when they had a good relationship with their therapist. Characteristics such as gender, age, and faith may affect how comfortable a patient feels with their therapist.

People experience anxiety differently, and effective treatment looks different for everyone. Someone may have to try several different therapists or types of therapy before they find one that works for them, and that's OK. Therapists genuinely want their patients to get better, even if that means referring them to a different therapist or recommending a different type of therapy.

Cognitive Behavioral Therapy

Cognitive behavioral therapy is one approach that has proven effective in treating anxiety. It differs from traditional psychotherapy in important ways. Traditional psychotherapies focus on events from the past that may have contributed to the present symptoms. In CBT the focus is on the present—identifying and changing unhealthy thought patterns or behaviors and contending with anxious thoughts or feelings as they crop up in daily life. Due to its focus on the present, CBT tends to be briefer and more effective than psychotherapies that focus mostly on the past.

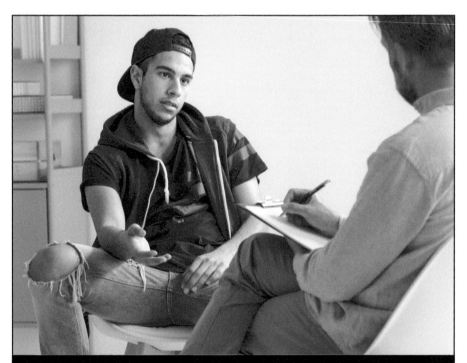

Research has shown that CBT can be effective in treating anxiety disorders, depression, substance use disorder, eating disorders, and other mental illnesses.

CBT is the combination of two treatment approaches—cognitive therapy and behavior therapy. Cognitive therapy uses strategies that help people change the unhealthy thinking patterns and beliefs behind their symptoms. Often this involves reframing beliefs or expectations about situations. The therapist may offer alternative ways of thinking about fear and fear responses. The therapist also helps people develop new, healthier thought patterns. This can reduce the frequency of anxious thoughts and shorten the length of time that a person spends dwelling on them when they occur. Behavior therapy helps people change the actions that maintain and worsen anxiety symptoms. It also gives patients strategies to actively manage their symptoms. Some very simple examples include taking deep breaths or placing one's hands on one's chest when feeling an anxiety spike. For anxiety disorders that deal with specific phobias, exposure-based behavior therapies can be very helpful.

COGNITIVE STRATEGIES

According to the principles of CBT, our world is not shaped by events or facts. Instead, our world is shaped by our value judgments of ourselves, about others, and about life. People with anxiety disorders tend to have an unrealistic, often irrationally high expectation that negative, even catastrophic, events are happening or about to happen. They have persistent feelings of doubt regarding their own or others' personal safety. They have negative thoughts that often begin with, "What if . . ." or "I should have. . . ." Some examples are these:

- "What if I'm having a heart attack?"
- "What if the airplane crashes?"

- "What if I get a life-threatening disease?"
- "What if I have a panic attack?"
- "What if I act upon this thought of harming my parents?"

Negative thoughts that cause anxiety are almost instantaneous and are often irrational. That's why some therapists refer to them as automatic thoughts. Behind these thoughts are faulty beliefs about self, others, and the world.

Cognitive strategies focus on discovering these faulty beliefs and then directly challenging and testing them. It can be very difficult and scary to challenge these faulty beliefs, especially when they have become such a large part of a person's way of viewing and interacting with the world. When automatic beliefs are challenged, often they turn out to be untrue. Once a person has challenged the faulty beliefs and the negative thoughts they breed, they can begin to replace them with more positive coping self-statements. Over time, this enables people to gain more and more control over automatic thoughts. Traditional practices like meditation emphasize that we can be unattached to our thoughts and that we can control our responses to our thoughts and feelings. Because of this, meditation practices and meditative behaviors have become a common strategy for managing anxious thoughts.

Challenging faulty beliefs is more than just positive thinking. It's better to call it accurate thinking. Through the process of therapy, dysfunctional beliefs and thoughts are tested, refuted, and replaced with more accurate and functional beliefs and thoughts. These functional beliefs and thoughts can help people interact with the world in a way that causes them less distress. Here are some faulty beliefs that are common among people with anxiety disorders:

- all-or-nothing thinking (black-and-white thinking)—
  "I'm a complete failure because I scored poorly on
  one test."
- overgeneralization (isolated negative events applied
  to all future events)—"She wouldn't go out with me.
  No one ever will!"
- mental filter (focusing on one negative detail)—"My
  weekend was completely ruined because we were
  late for the movie."
- mind reading (assuming others' negative opinions)—
  "My teacher must think I'm so bad at math."
- fortune-teller error/probability overestimation
  (predicting the future)—"I'll panic." "I'll freeze." "I'll
  definitely get sick and die."
- catastrophizing (assuming the worst)—"I have a
  headache. It certainly means I have cancer."
- emotional reasoning (feelings are the only
  evidence)—"I feel so foolish and uncool. I must really
  look foolish and uncool."
- "should" statements (unreasonably high
  standards)—"I should always be perfect, say the
  right thing, and be in perfect control all the time."
- personalization (arbitrary self-blame)—"My friend
  didn't smile at me in the hallway. I must have made
  her angry!"

In CBT, patients learn how to speak to themselves in healthier
ways. It could be compared to learning a new language—the
language of successfully coping with and managing fear. For
example, in CBT, people with panic disorder learn to interpret

51

physical symptoms differently. They replace the statement "My pulse is racing. I'm going to have a panic attack." Instead, they say to themselves, "My pulse is beating fast because I just walked up a flight of stairs." Or even, "My pulse is beating fast. It will likely slow down in a moment. It has in the past."

By using a new language, a person challenges their faulty beliefs about their anxiety. Some people who suffer from stage fright report that they are able to alleviate the physical symptoms of their stage fright by reframing the bodily sensations as their brain's

SCENARIO: Unexpected traffic on the way to school

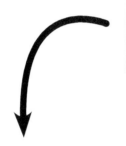

FAULTY BELIEF: I'm never going to make it to school on time.

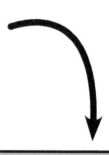

CHALLENGE THOUGHT: I may be late for school, but at least I'll get there safely.

attempt to protect them. Challenging faulty beliefs can help a person with PTSD identify self-blaming and shame-based beliefs that cause emotional pain and withdrawal. Challenging obsessive thoughts and faulty beliefs can help people with OCD resist their compulsive behaviors. Cognitive strategies aren't enough, however. For people with panic disorder, agoraphobia, OCD, specific phobias, and social phobia, the behavioral piece of cognitive behavioral therapy is especially important.

BEHAVIORAL STRATEGIES

Avoiding feared things, people, situations, or even thoughts actually sustain and reinforce anxiety. Exposure-based techniques are among the most effective behavioral strategies for helping people overcome avoidance. These techniques help people to gradually confront their fears by placing themselves in the situations they fear. In exposure and response prevention (ERP), also called ritual prevention, patients place themselves in the very situations that trigger fear. Exposure eventually reduces the anxiety and distress of fear-provoking situations through a natural process called habituation.

The nervous system naturally goes through habituation whenever it gets used to something that at first causes fear. Imagine easing yourself into a swimming pool filled with cold water. You sit on the edge of a pool and dip your foot into the cold water. It feels uncomfortably frigid. You want to immediately pull your foot out. But if you keep your foot in the water, after about thirty seconds, something changes. The water feels comfortable on your foot. Did the water temperature change? No. After prolonged exposure to the cold water, the temperature sensors in your skin got used to, or habituated to, the sensations of the cold water.

The technique of exposure uses this process of habituation to help people overcome phobias of all types. Imagine, for example, that you had never learned to swim. As a result, the very thought of getting within even a few feet of a swimming pool would be terrifying. Through the process of exposure, your fear could be overcome. You walk within a few feet of the swimming pool. You feel immediate discomfort. Your heart races, your stomach churns, your palms become sweaty, and your mouth becomes dry. After a few minutes, your fear starts to lessen as your nervous system habituates to the idea of being within a few feet of the dreaded swimming pool.

You now feel braver, so you inch closer to the pool's edge. Again, your fear rises and your heart races, your breathing pace increases, your hands get clammy, and you feel those butterflies in your

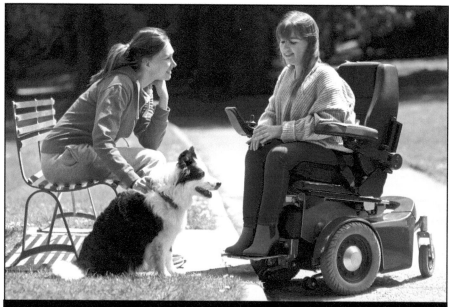

A person with a specific phobia of dogs may practice exposure therapy by spending time with a trusted friend's dog.

stomach. After a while, your fear again lessens as you habituate to the idea of being near the pool.

Determined to get into the pool, you then place one toe into the water, and once again the fear rises. But as before, after a few minutes, your nervous system habituates to the water. You submerge your ankle, then your calf, and then your knee. Slowly but gradually, you are in the water up to your waist, thanks to the capacity of your nervous system to adapt to the feared situation through habituation. You have mastered your fear through the use of your brain's natural alarm shut-off mechanism.

This is how exposure therapy works to help people overcome specific fears. A therapist will ask a person with an anxiety disorder to place themselves in direct contact with the things they fear. The approach is gradual, like moving slowly into the feared swimming pool. The ultimate goal is complete habituation to the feared object or situation. It's important to make certain that the exposure brings up the anxious feelings it's designed to help control. The idea is to experience the anxiety and realize that it can be tolerated and lessened without having to do the usual rituals or take other protective measures. For people with phobias, exposure means exposing oneself to feared items. For social phobia, it means exposure to feared social situations. People with panic disorder must gradually expose themselves to situations that trigger panic attacks.

Exposure to the physical sensations associated with the panic attacks may also be necessary. The therapist might assist the person in bringing on a rapid heart rate and heavy breathing, for example, and then help the person tolerate those feelings. With the help of an experienced therapist, imaginative exposure can help a person with post-traumatic stress disorder. Exposure to memories of the traumatic event is combined with cognitive strategies. The therapist helps the person move from "Memories are dangerous" to "I can recall without fear," from "The world is a dangerous place" to "I can cope," from "I am powerless" to "I have control," and from "I am incompetent" to "I can make good choices."

For people with PTSD, exposure to real-life situations that bring on anxiety can also be helpful. For example, a person might be avoiding certain areas, such as movie theaters, that bring on irrational fears. By going to movie theaters and not experiencing any negative or traumatic events, the person with PTSD can begin to lose their fear of such places.

For people with OCD, exposure is only half the story in ERP. The other important component, response prevention, means to actively and purposefully *not* do whatever the person usually feels compelled to do to relieve the immediate anxiety and discomfort of the obsessive thoughts. This may mean not washing hands, not checking door locks over and over, not counting, or not rethinking a thought "correctly." The idea is to allow the nervous system's natural habituation to lessen the anxiety of the thought, rather than trying to get anxiety relief through the compulsive behavior. This can be very difficult at first and may take many tries. This is normal and does not mean that the person will never get better. Eventually, the fear can be conquered.

During ERP, it's important to experience at least a moderate amount of anxiety and continue the exposure long enough for the anxiety to rise and then fall to manageable levels. When habituation occurs, nervous system boredom sets in. The mind has the chance to realize that the feared consequences, such as getting sick or burning the house down, aren't going to happen. When exposure is combined with response prevention, the brain can learn more appropriate reactions to the anxiety-provoking thoughts.

ERP can be highly challenging, especially for someone who is experiencing severe symptoms. (To address more severe symptoms, ERP should be pursued with a licensed therapist trained in this type of treatment.) Initially, someone can expect to feel very anxious as they confront anxiety-producing situations and block their learned habit of doing rituals in response to the anxiety.

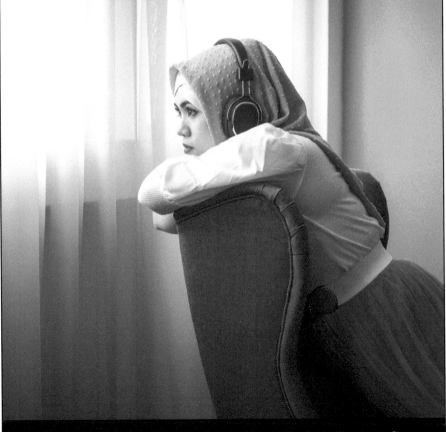

Listening to an imaginal exposure narrative can be extremely challenging at first. Over time, habituation can make intrusive thoughts less distressing.

At first, it may be too difficult to resist the ritual. A person with OCD might choose instead to delay the ritual or alter it in small ways, working gradually toward completely stopping. Sometimes it's almost impossible to do real-life exposure and response prevention because the fears involve events that could be impossible to re-create in the present. They might involve events that could possibly happen far off in the future—such as getting sick or causing a car accident. In these cases, imaginal exposure is useful. The patient describes a fear-provoking thought or idea in vivid detail and writes it down on paper as a moment-to-moment narrative. They record this three- to five-minute narrative on a phone or computer, play it back, and listen to it over and over until habituation occurs.

Treatment with ERP is hard work and requires patience and persistence to be successful. Even after the therapy ends, most people with OCD will need to continue using ERP principles, sometimes for the rest of their lives. Some may need to return to therapy for booster sessions to increase their ERP skills. While ERP principles are described in several self-help books, it's best to get started with a qualified mental health professional who is specifically trained in ERP for people with OCD. This is especially important for children and teens.

The Brain, Anxiety, and Medications

The brain is an incredibly intricate system of interconnected nerve cells, or neurons. These linked neurons form circuits that transmit messages in chemical form to all parts of the body. These messages help our bodies accomplish life-sustaining biological processes, including digestion, circulation, respiration, and our senses, among many others. Thinking, feeling, and behavior are also functions of this amazing system of interconnected circuits.

Neurotransmitters are brain chemicals that carry messages back and forth along these circuits. They bridge synapses—the tiny gaps between nerve cells. Imbalances in the levels of these neurotransmitters can severely disrupt the brain's regulation of biological processes. The imbalances can interrupt the circuits and the flow of chemical messages from one neuron to another. Neurons may send too many signals, or they may send too few. The brain may be overwhelmed with information, or it may not be receiving enough. This can result in psychiatric disorders, including anxiety disorders.

Three neurotransmitters appear to play major roles in anxiety disorders: serotonin, norepinephrine, and gamma-aminobutyric acid (GABA). Norepinephrine can activate the fight-or-flight response, while GABA and serotonin have a calming effect. Serotonin is vital to the brain's capacity to regulate moods properly. People with anxiety disorders can have imbalances of these neurotransmitters. They may have too much norepinephrine, sending their nervous system into constant overdrive as it prepares for danger. Or they

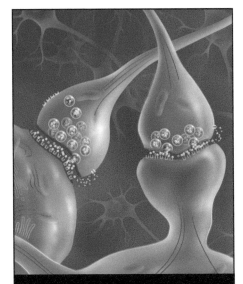

Neurotransmitters (yellow and blue dots) cross the gaps between neurons, called synapses, and are essential to the function of complex neural systems. Scientists have identified more than five hundred different types of neurotransmitters in the human body.

may be lacking in GABA or serotonin, making it much harder for the brain to wind down and relax. Certain medications correct these imbalances, reducing the person's anxiety symptoms.

Antidepressants can be highly effective in treating anxiety disorders. These medications are called selective serotonin reuptake inhibitors, or SSRIs. Doctors commonly recommend and prescribe SSRIs such as fluoxetine (Prozac), fluvoxamine (Luvox), paroxetine (Paxil), sertraline (Zoloft), citalopram (Celexa), venlafaxine (Effexor), and escitalopram oxalate (Lexapro). They work for people with anxiety disorders by increasing the amount of serotonin at the brain's synapses. The chemical bridges the gaps between nerve cells so that chemical messages can flow more effectively. The result is a significant reduction in anxiety symptoms—and in depression symptoms for patients who also have depression.

The medications are non-habit forming and have far fewer side effects than older antianxiety medications. All SSRIs work in similar ways, but each is somewhat different. Depending on the disorder, SSRIs may take four to eight weeks to achieve a positive result. Sometimes the first medication a patient uses won't relieve anxiety well enough. A doctor will then prescribe a different SSRI. Sometimes a patient will need to try several before finding one that works well. Occasionally, other medications are prescribed along with SSRIs to help relieve anxiety.

Many anxiety disorders are affected by the neurotransmitter GABA. Because of this, doctors sometimes prescribe medications that affect GABA. These drugs are called benzodiazepines. The ones doctors most commonly recommend are alprazolam (Xanax), clonazepam (Klonopin), diazepam (Valium), and lorazepam (Ativan). Benzodiazepines are most appropriate for short-term treatment.

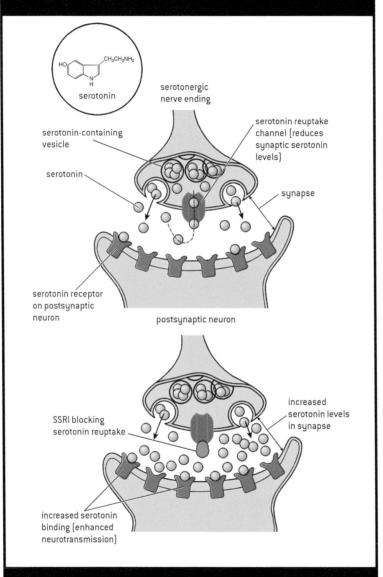

HOW SSRIS WORK

serotonin

serotonergic nerve ending

serotonin-containing vesicle

serotonin reuptake channel (reduces synaptic serotonin levels)

serotonin

synapse

serotonin receptor on postsynaptic neuron

postsynaptic neuron

SSRI blocking serotonin reuptake

increased serotonin levels in synapse

increased serotonin binding (enhanced neurotransmission)

SSRIs block some of the reuptake receptors in neurons to increase synaptic neurotransmitter levels. More neurotransmitters in the synapses make it easier to transmit messages between neurons.

ANXIETY DISORDERS AND MINORITY POPULATIONS

For a long time, the instance of anxiety disorders was thought to be greatest among white populations. A study published in 2009 found that rates of anxiety disorders were also significant among Black and Hispanic populations. Additionally, severity of mental illness in these populations was higher than among their white counterparts. Some of this may have to do with stressors that are specific to or more common in minority populations, such as institutional racism, economic instability, and exposure to violent crime. According to the Health and Human Services Office of Minority Health, Black Americans are 20 percent more likely than the general population to suffer from serious mental health problems. For example, Black Americans experience PTSD at a higher rate than any other racial group.

Marginalized communities can face significant barriers to support and treatment. Availability and accessibility are two major factors. A person with inadequate health insurance coverage may be unable to afford the services and medications they need. Someone may have to travel a significant distance to reach a clinic or take time off work to make an appointment. At the clinic, language barriers may exist for those who speak a language other than English.

There is also a history of improper treatment for minority communities in health care, due in part to biases reinforced in medical school and postgraduate training. For many decades, medical study participants were limited to white men and women. As a result, students are mostly taught to identify disorders in white patients. However, these disorders can present differently in patients of color, and doctors run the risk of misdiagnosis. The biases learned by older doctors are then reinforced in the next generation of doctors during residency training. There is a large movement in the health-care community to address racial bias in medicine. Many professionals are working to change educational practices and institute more equitable policies and practices in diagnosis and treatment. Nevertheless, some people who find the courage to come forward about their symptoms may be misdiagnosed, and their treatment may be further complicated by conscious or unconscious bias from their medical provider. It is important for someone experiencing an anxiety disorder to find a therapist who can empathize with their specific identity experiences. This can lead to better outcomes and more effective treatment. A good resource for finding an appropriate therapist is www.adaa.org.

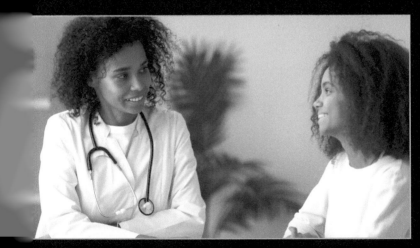

Culturally competent health-care providers integrate individual factors such as race, ethnicity, gender, socioeconomic status, and sexual orientation into their patients' treatment plans.

ANXIETY DISORDERS AND DEPRESSION

Many people with OCD and other anxiety disorders suffer from depressive symptoms. These range from mild to severe, life-threatening depressive illness characterized by strong, persistent feelings of sadness, hopelessness, helplessness, loss of interest in normal activities and pursuits, lack of energy, impaired sleep and appetite, and suicidal thoughts. If anxiety is a problem for you or someone you know, keep a lookout for signs of major depressive disorder. These include the following:

- depressed mood most of the day, nearly every day
- diminished interest or pleasure in all or almost all activities
- significant weight loss or gain, or decrease or increase in appetite nearly every day
- insomnia or excessive sleep nearly every day
- feelings of extreme restlessness or of being slowed down
- fatigue or loss of energy nearly every day
- feelings of worthlessness or excessive or inappropriate guilt nearly every day
- diminished ability to think or concentrate, or indecisiveness, nearly every day
- recurrent thoughts of death or of suicide without a specific plan
- a plan for attempting suicide or an actual attempt

They work quickly, so patients sometimes take them until their prescribed SSRI achieves its full benefit. They are, however, habit-forming, so the body can become dependent on them. Doctors tend to avoid prescribing these medications for long-term use, and they take special care when stopping them. Abrupt withdrawal can produce panic attacks, confusion, severe anxiety, muscle tension, irritability, insomnia, and seizures.

Other antidepressants are also used to treat anxiety disorders, especially in the few cases when SSRIs are not effective. For example, another class of medications, called beta-blockers, can be helpful for reducing the physical symptoms of anxiety, such as rapid or irregular heartbeats, sweating, shaking, and tremors. The two that doctors most commonly prescribe are atenolol (Tenormin) and propranolol (Inderal). They have been used effectively to reduce the symptoms associated with stage fright, a common social phobia.

Medication can be an important part of treating an anxiety disorder. But medication alone rarely eliminates all the symptoms. A well-rounded treatment plan includes CBT and medication. Some people with mild or moderate anxiety disorders can be effectively treated without medication. Additionally, some people who try medication report unwelcome side effects such as grogginess or fogginess, a feeling of disconnect, and effects on sexual desire. Someone taking a medication should always take it according to the instructions, but if they do not like their current medication, they can speak with a doctor about stopping or switching medications. Many people will have a negative reaction to one medication but will not experience these same side effects after switching to another medication. A doctor can help someone safely explore medications to find the right one for them.

Are Medications for Anxiety Disorders Safe?

In October 2004, the United States Food and Drug Administration (FDA) issued a warning that SSRIs may increase suicidal thoughts and behaviors in a small number of children and adolescents. The

EMERGENCY HELPLINES

The Substance Abuse and Mental Health Services Administration offers a free hotline at 800-662-4357. People can call when a crisis occurs such as an anxiety attack or panic attack. Their trained responders are available twenty-four hours a day and can provide judgment-free support and resources.

The National Suicide Prevention Lifeline is a toll-free hotline in the US for people who are in distress and at risk of harming themselves. The service has a network of over 160 crisis centers across the country. Anyone can call the lifeline at 800-273-8255 and connect with a trained crisis worker at their nearest crisis center. Conversations are confidential, and workers are trained to be active, nonjudgmental listeners. They can also provide resources to callers concerned about a friend or family member.

For those who prefer to communicate by text, the Crisis Text Line is a free and confidential service where trained crisis counselors provide support. The text line is available through Facebook Messenger, WhatsApp, and text message at 741741.

These resources are intended to help people before they act on suicidal thoughts. If you or someone you know has a plan for suicide, call 911 immediately.

FDA report was based on a review of twenty-four short-term studies (four to sixteen weeks long) of nine antidepressant medications, including SSRIs. The studies involved more than forty-four hundred children and adolescents with major depressive disorder, obsessive-compulsive disorder, and other psychiatric disorders. Analyses of the studies showed that, on average, 4 percent of patients treated with an antidepressant developed suicidal ideation or suicidal behaviors, compared to 2 percent of patients who were given a placebo (sugar pill). A suicide did not occur in any of the studies.

The FDA warning did not prohibit the use of these medications in children and adolescents. The FDA notes that the small risk of suicidal thoughts and behaviors must be balanced with the clinical need for the medications for each individual child. For the vast majority of children with anxiety disorders, these medications are safe and effective.

While the risks of taking SSRIs are extremely small, doctors and caregivers carefully monitor children and teens taking these medications. For the first few months after a patient starts using an antidepressant, doctors watch for changes in the patient's behavior, including agitation, restlessness, and irritability. If these changes occur, the patient's doctor can adjust the dose or change medications. There are a lot of different SSRIs, which can be used in different dosages and combinations, and not all of them have the same side effects. Patients should never just stop taking their medication abruptly without their doctor's supervision since this may worsen symptoms.

CHAPTER FOUR

STRESS MANAGEMENT

In addition to cognitive behavioral therapy and medications, therapists often recommend lifestyle changes to relieve anxiety and distress. These lifestyle changes can help manage the stress of daily living. Everyone can benefit from stress management tools.

Almost any change, positive or negative, causes stress. Stress is not necessarily bad. Stress prompts the brain's fight-or-flight response, part of a range of biological responses that are essential to successfully facing life's challenges, including change. Some responses are turned on for a long time, especially in situations involving major changes that feel unpredictable and uncontrollable—like illness, divorce, sudden trauma, or financial hardship. These responses take a toll on the body. Excessive stress can contribute to heart disease, high blood pressure, diabetes, headaches, ulcers, chronic diarrhea, muscle tension, and many other physical ailments.

Living with excessive stress can severely challenge a person's capacity to cope and can potentially result in chronic psychological and physical problems. Even moderate or low-level stress can have a negative impact on our bodies if it is sustained over time.

Since stress can have a negative impact on our bodies, people need breaks from stress. The goal isn't to eliminate all stress. Positive stress, or eustress, can help to make life rewarding and full. Examples of eustress are exercise, cheering a favorite team, and getting together with friends. The goals are to eliminate distress, add eustress, and take breaks from stress.

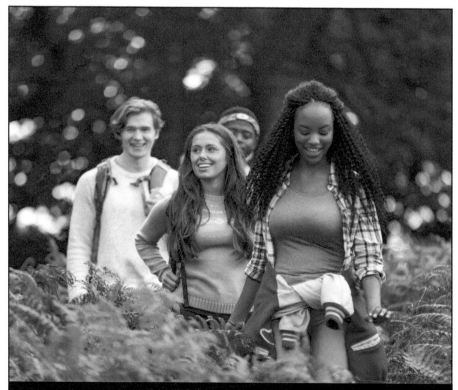

Many people find spending time in nature improves their mental health.

What do you consider stressful? This can be different for everyone. Events such as failing an important test, moving to a new school, getting arrested, or breaking up with a significant other may generate extreme feelings of stress or anxiety. Someone else may consider them only a challenge or as just a part of everyday life. Stress comes when your brain perceives something as a threat to your physical or psychological well-being and believes that the threat can't be coped with. Events do not cause stress. Instead, it is the *perception* of those events, and the learned beliefs about them, that result in stress and anxiety. When you notice signs of stress in your body—such as nervousness, anger, worry, headaches, back pain, and indigestion—stop and take a deep breath or two. Observe your negative thoughts. Is there a more positive way of looking at the stress-causing situation? Can you see it as a challenge or an opportunity for growth? Can you see the humor in the situation? Multiple studies have shown that it is more difficult to experience stress while you are smiling or laughing.

If the worry is caused by something serious—such as illness or death—look for ways to share and manage your burden by involving others. Talk to a trusted friend, family member, or other adult. Ask for help. You can look for a trusted adult at school, at your church, or in an after-school activity. Even during times of low stress, work to build and grow a network of support so it will be there when needed.

If worry is a problem, saying to yourself, "Stop worrying!" just doesn't work. For people who are not experiencing a severe anxiety disorder, it can feel helpful to schedule ten to thirty minutes every day for worrying so that your worry is not bothering you all day long. The best time is toward the end of the day, when you've likely collected some things to worry about. Don't make it so late in the day that you're feeling tired. Fatigue can increase worry and anxiety, and it can disrupt sleep patterns.

The trick is to limit yourself to worrying only during the chosen time. When worries pop up before your worry time, write them down on a "Worry List" to get them out of your mind until later in the day. This way, instead of saying "Stop," you're saying "Wait." During your worry time, do nothing but worry. When your mind wanders, bring it back to worrying. The important thing is to postpone worry the rest of the day so that constant worry does not interfere with your other activities. If you find that this is difficult or you are experiencing physical symptoms of anxiety during this worry time, reach out to a trusted person or health-care provider and ask for help.

In addition, you can cut down on your worries by getting more organized. Establish clear goals with plans to achieve those goals. Prepare for the next day and the next week by making lists, keeping a planner, or using a scheduling app. Divide large tasks into smaller, more manageable steps. Plan small breaks and rewards for yourself to motivate you to power through long or difficult tasks. This can help you feel more in control of your daily life and less overwhelmed.

While many things are out of our control, we often worry about things we can actually do something about. Ask yourself if you can do anything about a specific worry on your list. Write down all the options that come to mind, and then choose a plan of action. Write down the steps you'll take to address the problem and then carry out the plan. If it doesn't work, choose another plan. Consult with trusted friends, family members, or advisers. You may find that simply talking through your problems with a willing listener can relieve a significant amount of stress. But talking about a problem over and over can stop being helpful and begin to increase stress. If so, give yourself a break from discussing the problem until you have a new idea about a possible solution.

Relaxation

Taking time for relaxing activities, such as listening to music, reading books for pleasure, talking with friends, and reflecting on spiritual matters gives our minds and bodies breaks from negative stress. Recreational activities, community involvement, and exercise can provide positive eustress that helps build emotional, mental, and physical resilience. If we fill our lives with too many activities, they begin to add too much stress. Balance is key to effective stress management. Two or three yoga sessions a week might be relaxing. Doing yoga twice a day, however, might begin to take so much time away from other activities that it becomes stressful.

Another technique, the relaxation response, is a form of relaxation that has a profound physical effect on the body. Relaxation response—the opposite of stress response—was first described by the medical doctor Herbert Benson in the 1970s. It refers to a state of deep relaxation when heart rate, respiration, blood pressure, and muscle tension are all decreased. Using relaxation techniques to induce a state of deep relaxation is an option for people who need to give their bodies a break from excess stress. It can reduce anxiety and fatigue, increase energy, and improve productivity, memory, and concentration.

Spending twenty to thirty minutes a day in a state of relaxation helps reduce stress during the rest of the day. With practice, a person can also relax more easily throughout the day, reducing their stress even more. The most common techniques include progressive muscle relaxation, abdominal breathing, visualization, meditation, guided imagery, and biofeedback. An easy and effective relaxation exercise is to observe and change your breathing pattern. When people are anxious, they tend to breathe more shallowly and rapidly from the chest. Relaxed breathing, however, is slower and deeper and is centered in the abdomen. All of these activities focus on breath. Deep breathing can help to stimulate the vagus nerve, a long nerve that runs from the brain to the abdomen, and trigger the body's natural relaxation response. Many people are turning to breath work or yoga for help with stress management.

Take a few moments to observe your breathing right now. Sit or lie down with your hand placed on your abdomen, just below your ribs. Does your abdomen expand when you inhale? Relax your abdominal muscles, and breathe in slowly and deeply through your nose so that your abdomen rises. Pause, and then exhale slowly and completely through your nose. Your hand on your abdomen should

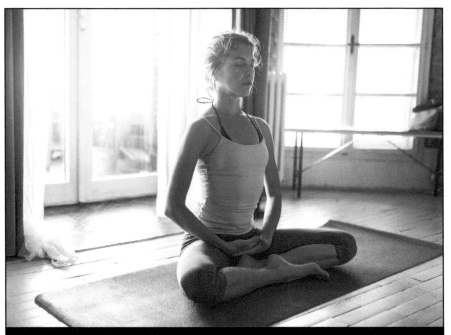

Yoga incorporates both physical and mental disciplines to help achieve peacefulness in body and mind.

go up as you inhale and down as you exhale. Breathe in, pause, and breathe out. Do this gently, slowly, and smoothly about ten times. After practicing abdominal breathing daily at home, you'll find it easier to transition into a more relaxed breathing pattern when you find yourself breathing anxiously from your chest.

Many apps and online videos—some of which are free— offer coaching in breath work. These resources may differ in the background noise they offer, the amount of time they suggest practicing for, or the spacing and timing of breath. The range of resources available can allow people to experiment with different techniques until they discover what works best for them.

Take Care of Your Body

The human mind and body are closely connected. Being aware of this relationship can help a person manage anxiety. For example, a healthy diet can reduce anxiety and stress. If making a huge change to your diet is intimidating or anxiety provoking, start with just a few healthier eating habits and build on your success gradually. A stress-reducing diet is well balanced and high in fruits and vegetables. It's low in refined carbohydrates—foods such as potato chips, white bread, cakes, pies, and candy. But there's plenty of room for complex carbohydrates, such as whole grain bread and cereals, brown rice, and vegetables. A stress-reducing diet is also low in saturated fats such as butter or coconut oil. Healthier sources of fat are nuts and monounsaturated oils—olive and canola oils, for example. Healthy sources of protein include fish, beans, soy products, and legumes. This type of diet is good for your heart and brain. Being too worried about eating the "right" foods can also cause stress. Balance is important. A sweet treat or a bag of potato chips once in a while can be fun. A hamburger with friends or a piece of birthday cake with your family can be a relaxing way to connect with the people you care about! Of course, eating only birthday cake and hamburgers every day would exacerbate symptoms of stress and anxiety by causing a spike in blood sugar and by increasing stress hormone levels. But in moderation, any food that your body isn't allergic to or intolerant of is fine to eat and enjoy.

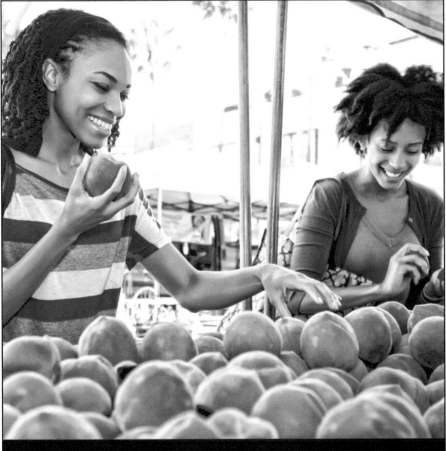

A balanced diet can help you to feel your best, both mentally and physically.

Avoid Stimulants

Some foods and beverages can make anxiety worse. Caffeine has a stimulating effect, for example, and produces the same effects as stress on the body, such as increased heart rate, shallow breathing, and increased perspiration. Some caffeine can help focus the body, but too much may have the opposite effect, causing feelings of jitteriness or panic. Cutting back or eliminating caffeine can reduce restlessness, irritability, and difficulty sleeping.

Caffeine can be found in coffee, tea, soda, chocolate, and some over-the-counter medications. Abrupt withdrawal from caffeine may cause headache, fatigue, and depression. Most people find it easier to taper off caffeine gradually. It may take a while to adapt to life without caffeine or with reduced caffeine, but the body will eventually adjust and get back to normal.

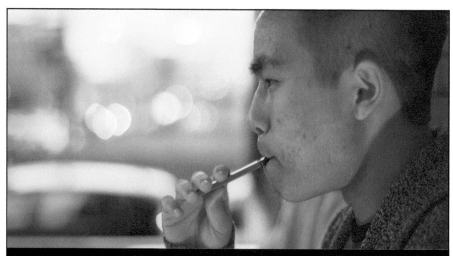

Nicotine has been shown to impact impulse control, particularly in young adults. It can also affect one's ability to learn and pay attention by altering developing neurons in the brain.

Nicotine is also a stimulant. Some people claim that smoking or vaping is relaxing. This may be due to the physical action of inhaling and exhaling. Focusing on the breath and breathing deeply is a very effective relaxation technique, but the body's physical response to nicotine is the opposite of relaxation. While quitting smoking or vaping can be stressful, the long-term result is stress reduction and a healthier body.

Some nonprescription and prescription medications contain stimulants and may also increase anxiety. Pseudoephedrine, often found in cold and allergy medications, can leave you feeling restless and nervous. Alcohol and other drugs can have varying effects from person to person. What might relax one individual may cause anxiety in another. Strong stimulants such as ephedra, amphetamines, and cocaine are especially dangerous for people at risk for panic attacks and anxiety disorders.

Exercise

Physical exercise is an example of the eustress that we need in our lives. Exercise stimulates the production of endorphins, natural pain-reducing and mood-moderating chemicals. Exercise enhances oxygenation of the blood and brain. With more oxygen in the blood and brain, we are better able to concentrate, remember things, and remain alert. Exercise also reduces muscle tension, improves blood circulation and digestion, and reduces blood pressure.

Exercise can be especially helpful for people with depression and anxiety disorders. People with panic disorder sometimes avoid exercise that raises their heart rate. They fear that increasing their heart rate might trigger a panic attack. Gradually increasing the amount or intensity of exercise along with challenging faulty beliefs about normal heartbeat acceleration can help people with panic disorder benefit

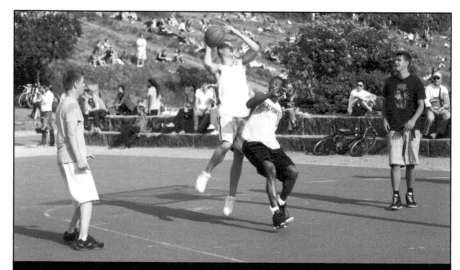

A regular game of pickup basketball with friends can make exercise something to look forward to.

from exercise. They will gradually feel less fearful of the physical aspects of panic attacks. Aerobic exercise is a good option for reducing stress, anxiety, and muscle tension. It also improves cardiovascular fitness. Aerobic exercise is any physical activity that raises heart rate and increases the efficiency of oxygen intake by the body. This type of exercise includes running, brisk walking, swimming, cycling, and dancing. Anaerobic exercise involves short bursts of activity and builds muscle. Examples include weight lifting and short-distance swimming or sprinting. Yoga is another form of exercise that can be beneficial. It focuses on moving the body intentionally and staying in touch with breath. Yoga has been studied in clinical trials with anxiety and depression due to its relaxing and grounding effects. In these studies, yoga has been shown to help people experiencing anxiety and depression feel more connected to their bodies and their breath and to help reduce symptoms of anxiety and depression.

The most beneficial kind of exercise is the kind that you enjoy and that you can keep up consistently. Most doctors recommend twenty to thirty minutes of exercise four to five times a week, and it's OK to miss one or two of those days if it's a tough week. If your body and mind are under a lot of stress, it may be more beneficial to take a day off and get some rest! The overall pattern is what is most important for staying healthy.

Gentle movement can also help to manage stress. Exercise doesn't have to be high intensity. The American Heart Association recommends taking ten thousand steps a day for optimal health. Taking a walk through the neighborhood as part of your morning routine, during lunch, or after the school or workday can be a very effective way of caring for your body and clearing your mind. Maybe invite a friend along so that you can reap the stress-reducing benefits of gentle exercise and companionship together!

Rest and Laughter

In addition to nourishment and exercise, the body needs rest. Sleep provides rest and rejuvenation for the brain, the mind, and the body. Inadequate sleep has a negative effect on the neurotransmitters GABA and serotonin. This causes anxiety and stress, making it even more difficult to sleep. The best way to avoid this cycle is to maintain good sleep habits. Everyone needs a different amount of sleep, but the general recommended amount of sleep is seven to nine hours every night. Children and adolescents should aim for about eight to ten hours of sleep each night. Being tired or sleepy during the day, having an overwhelming desire to take a nap, or not being as alert as usual are all signs that someone probably needs more sleep than they are getting. Some helpful tips to improve sleeping habits are trying to get up and go to bed at the same time every day and going to bed at a moderate level of tiredness. Waiting too long to go to sleep can create stress and overstimulation, which can make it harder to fall asleep.

Develop a relaxing bedtime routine by reducing noise, light, stimulation, and activity before bed. Avoid caffeine in the evening, as well as alcohol. Alcohol may seem relaxing, but it actually disrupts sleep patterns. So does watching television, looking at computer screens, and scrolling social media. If possible, get computers and cell phones out of the room at night. A light snack before bed can be helpful. Regular exercise improves sleep, but it is important to complete the routine at least a few hours before bedtime. Exercising too close to bedtime can increase the body's wakefulness system and make it more difficult to unwind and fall asleep. When unable to fall asleep, try getting up and doing something relaxing—such as reading or listening to quiet music—in another room. Keep in mind that screen time does not count as a relaxing activity in this case.

Our minds and bodies need more rest than what we get from sleep. Setting aside time daily for relaxing activities can also help rest and rejuvenate the mind. Try to take an extended break every week for rest and recreation, and periodically take a vacation. A vacation can be two weeks visiting family, a week at a theme park or camp, or several days relaxing and hanging out with friends before the start of a new school year. Don't stop there, though. At the first sign of stress in your body, take a mini-break. Some options are taking a short walk, standing up and stretching, or calling a family member or friend. Slightly longer breaks, such as an evening to yourself, going to the coffee shop with a book, cooking yourself a delicious and nutritious meal, or taking the morning to lie in bed

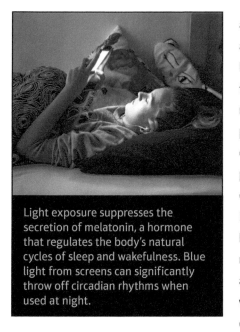

Light exposure suppresses the secretion of melatonin, a hormone that regulates the body's natural cycles of sleep and wakefulness. Blue light from screens can significantly throw off circadian rhythms when used at night.

and journal, can help you relax and reset before or after a busy day. Some people also find certain activities to be relaxing. For example, some people experience states of deep relaxation when knitting, playing a musical instrument, drawing, or playing video games. If you have a hobby that you love and that makes you feel more relaxed and calm, it can be a very good resource for coping with stress. If you don't have a current hobby that helps reduce stress, try one out! It's never too late to learn something new.

Perhaps the ultimate rest for the body and mind is humor. Laughter has been proven to decrease stress. It can temporarily lift anxiety and depression and help us connect with others. More important, humor and laughter help us perceive life differently. Seeing the humor in situations makes those situations less threatening and lowers our stress. If you need to relax, consider talking to your funniest friend, watching a funny movie, or looking up video clips of comedians.

Set Goals

Stress sometimes comes from feeling unfulfilled. Finding a sense of purpose and working toward achieving goals can help. Having well-defined goals and plans reduces stress. Take a moment to list your short-term goals: things you'd like to achieve today or in the next few weeks or months. Then list your long-term goals: things you'd like to achieve during your lifetime. Next, list ideas from this chapter that can help you reduce negative stress. You'll find that many of them will also help you achieve some of your goals.

Some people are stressed out by the thought of setting goals or worry that they won't reach them. It's OK to start small. Pick some goals you know you can accomplish, such as "eat breakfast," "walk the dog," or "make the bed." Making and achieving smaller goals can help you build confidence in your ability to meet your longer-term goals.

Anxiety and Stress Relief: What *Doesn't* Work

For many reasons, people often try other methods to relieve anxiety and stress. Some of these methods seem harmless. But they may keep a person from trying measures that are more effective. Some attempts to relieve anxiety and stress can be dangerous, even life-threatening. Below is a list of some of the ineffective ways people try to cope with anxiety and stress. All of these measures are very common. Almost everyone has engaged or knows someone who has engaged in one or many of these behaviors.

STRESS EATING

Eating unhealthy foods, eating too much, or eating too little all cause stress in the body and mind. Some people overeat when they're under stress, while others practically stop eating. Many treat themselves to comfort foods such as chips and ice cream and other desserts when they're upset or under stress. While it is OK to have a treat every once in a while, too many unhealthy foods can aggravate stress levels by increasing blood sugar and stress hormone levels. It can be helpful to plan ahead, substitute healthier foods for comfort foods the majority of the time, and make sure you are eating enough to fuel your body and your daily activities. Using food or lack of food to cope with stress can eventually turn into something more serious. If you suspect that you or someone you know might be dealing with an eating disorder, it is important to get help as soon as possible. These disorders can be very dangerous, but recovery is possible and easier the sooner the person gets help.

EXCESSIVE SHOPPING, INTERNET SURFING, GAMBLING, AND OTHER BEHAVIORS

Shopping, playing video games, surfing the internet, texting, watching TV, and many other activities can be relaxing in reasonable doses. But anything done to excess can lead people to overlook important chores, perform poorly at school or at work, spend too much money, or ignore important relationships. When this happens, the activity becomes stressful—even addictive—rather than relaxing. Using positive stress management skills can help reduce the likelihood of relying on excessive or addictive activities to relieve stress and anxiety. If you or someone you know is experiencing addiction to one or any of these activities, seek help. When engaging in a behavior disrupts other aspects of your life, no matter what that behavior is, a licensed therapist or counselor may be able to help you or your loved one rebalance their priorities.

GETTING ANGRY

Sometimes a person experiences stress when emotions such as anger, resentment, and jealousy toward others aren't expressed directly or appropriately. Suppressing these emotions can result in increased distress, moodiness, and even depression. On the other hand, giving free rein to these emotions in the form of rants, tantrums, aggressive behavior, bullying, or risk-taking can be destructive and even dangerous. It is important to learn to communicate painful feelings honestly, directly, and respectfully with others. It can be a great stress reliever. For help with this, it is best to seek the confidential guidance of a mental health counselor who is trained in working with young people. A counselor can help someone get in touch with feelings and express them appropriately.

ISOLATION

Taking an occasional break from the stress and pressures of daily life is an important part of maintaining emotional health and well-being. But it's unhealthy to completely stop devoting time to friends, family, and usual activities; to sleep more than usual for long stretches of time; or to miss school, work, and other obligations. When this is happening, there could be a problem. Social withdrawal is one of the symptoms of depression, which is common among teens and adults with anxiety disorders.

ALCOHOL AND DRUG USE

People drink or use drugs for many reasons. They may see it as a way to relieve boredom and loneliness. Others may feel pressure to seem cool or to fit in. They may also be trying to cope with negative feelings such as anxiety, fear, depression, grief, frustration, anger, shame, and guilt. At first, alcohol or drugs may seem to relieve these unpleasant emotions. Experimental and recreational use of drugs and alcohol may appear harmless when done on occasion. Under the right circumstances, however, a persistent pattern of use and eventual misuse—including substance use disorder—can develop. Besides the risk of dependence, other costs of alcohol and drug use include these:

- being arrested for possession of illegal drugs, driving while under the influence of alcohol or drugs (DUI), and other substance use–related offenses
- impaired ability to drive or operate machinery
- temporary physical discomfort after substance use, such as headache, stomachache, vomiting, and dizziness
- worsening of an existing anxiety disorder, depression, or physical disorder
- interference with school, work, and social life
- sleep difficulties
- added stress after the high is over, since the problems that were present before the high do not go away
- short-term memory loss and overall loss of motivation
- alienation from family and friends
- financial difficulties

Many risks are associated with drug and alcohol use. For teens, alcohol and illegal drugs carry additional costs because their use is illegal. Arrests create stress and stigma that can last a lifetime. For those with anxiety disorders, drugs or alcohol may make the condition worse and make it harder to seek effective medical treatment.

YOU CAN MANAGE AN ANXIETY DISORDER

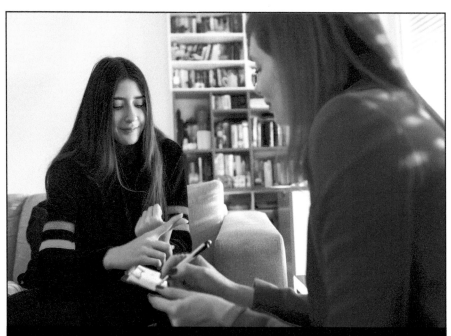

Individualized treatment plans that include therapy, medication, or both can significantly improve health outcomes for people living with anxiety disorders.

Being diagnosed with an anxiety disorder can feel devastating. Someone with an anxiety disorder may fear that they will have to live their whole life with anxiety, fear, worry, or depression. It doesn't have to be this way. By partnering with a mental health professional, people can find anxiety management strategies that work for them, from therapy to medication to lifestyle changes or a combination of these approaches. Many people have experienced severe anxiety disorders, sought treatment, and are then able to live healthy, fulfilling lives. Even people who aren't experiencing a severe anxiety disorder can learn and master stress management skills, such as the ones in this book, and emerge healthier and able to cope better with the challenges of life.

CELEBRITIES AND MENTAL HEALTH MANAGEMENT

Many celebrities have opened up about their own struggles with mental health and about the tactics and resources they have used to manage it.

- Actor and musician Selena Gomez has spoken out about her struggle with her mental health over her career, as well as her struggle with the autoimmune condition lupus. She said that she relies heavily on regular meetings with her therapist as well as dialectical behavior therapy to manage her depression, anxiety, and bipolar disorder. Gomez said that dialectical behavior therapy changed her life. In April 2021, Gomez announced a new campaign called Mental Health 101 to support mental health education and mental health services. "I know how scary and lonely it can feel to face anxiety and depression by yourself at a young age," she wrote in an Instagram post. "If I had learned about my mental health earlier on—been taught about my condition in school the way I was taught about other subjects—my journey would have looked very different. The world needs to know that mental health matters."

- Author John Green has been open about his struggles with OCD and anxiety throughout his career. The main character of his book *Turtles All the Way Down* grapples with similar mental health disorders. "It was really hard, especially at first, to write about this thing that's been such a big part of my life," he said in an interview in 2017. "But in another way, it was really empowering because I felt like if I could give it form or expression I could look at it and I could talk about it directly rather than being scared of it." He hopes that writing about mental illness for young adults will help to further destigmatize it.

- In 2019 singer Ariana Grande shared a brain scan of her brain on social media. She experienced severe PTSD after a bomb killed twenty-two people during her 2017 concert in Manchester, England. While she hasn't publicly discussed the exact treatment she's received, she's known for relying on the emotional support of her dogs to help her calm down. In June 2021, Grande announced a new partnership with BetterHelp, a digital therapy app, to give away $2 million in therapy sessions. "I so hope that this will be a helpful starting point," she wrote in an Instagram post announcing the partnership. "Healing is not linear or easy but you are worth the effort and time, I promise!"

- Professional basketball player Marcus Morris talked about his struggles with depression and anxiety, and especially about the interplay of race and mental health. He began seeing a psychologist in 2018. Since then, he has been an advocate for professional athletes to talk about and seek help for their mental health.

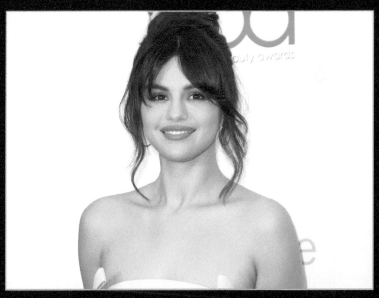

Selena Gomez has spoken candidly about her mental health and uses her platform to raise awareness for mental health issues.

GLOSSARY

acute stress disorder: a psychiatric disorder characterized by distressing psychological and physical symptoms following exposure to a traumatic event. The symptoms subside in less than one month.

adrenaline: also called epinephrine, a hormone produced by the adrenal gland in response to stress. Together with norepinephrine, it causes an increase in heart rate, blood pressure, mental activity, blood flow to the muscles, and metabolism. This prepares a person to deal with stress or perceived threats.

agoraphobia: an extreme fear of being in open or public places; a psychiatric disorder in which a person's fear results in the avoidance of many situations and places that the person considers to be unsafe

antidepressants: medications that are designed to ease the symptoms of depressive illness. They are also known to relieve the symptoms of various anxiety disorders.

anxiety: an excessive, out-of-proportion response to a vague, ill-defined, future-oriented threat. It is often accompanied by physiological signs, doubt about the reality and nature of the threat, and self-doubt about one's ability to cope with the threat.

anxiety disorder: a psychiatric disorder in which anxiety is the predominant symptom

benzodiazepines: a group of medications that produce calming effects by enhancing the action of the neurotransmitter gamma-aminobutyric acid

circadian rhythms: physical, mental, and behavioral changes that follow a twenty-four hour cycle

cognitive behavioral therapy (CBT): a psychologically based therapy that includes strategies for helping people modify behavior and change dysfunctional beliefs that sustain anxiety and depressive symptoms

cognitive strategies: therapeutic techniques that focus on identifying faulty automatic beliefs and the negative thoughts that result from them and then directly challenging and testing them. Further techniques are used to replace them with accurate, positive, and functional beliefs and thoughts.

compulsions: repetitive behaviors or mental acts, often performed in an effort to diminish or neutralize the anxiety and distress brought on by the obsessive thoughts of obsessive-compulsive disorder

depression: an emotional state characterized by persistent and strong feelings of sadness, helplessness, and hopelessness; crying or frequent tearfulness; lack of energy; loss of interest in normal activities and pursuits; impaired appetite; weight loss or gain; impaired sleep; and suicidal feelings or thoughts

dialectical behavior therapy: a type of CBT that combines strategies like mindfulness, emotional regulation, and healthy relationship management

distress: mental or physical strain brought about by pain, trouble, or worry; negative stress that is a result of a negative event in a person's life

dopamine: a neurotransmitter that is involved in the control of movement and the sensation of pleasure

eustress: positive stress that is a result of a positive event in a person's life

exposure and response prevention (ERP): also called exposure and response ritual prevention, a behavior therapy technique in which a person confronts a feared situation by doing the actions or thinking the thoughts that create discomfort or fear. Meanwhile, the patient is required to refrain from doing the usual behavioral ritual employed to reduce the discomfort.

fear: a feeling of agitation and apprehension as a response to a well-defined danger, a specific object, or a particular situation

fight-or-flight response: a set of specific physiological changes, such as elevated heart rate and blood pressure, shortness of breath, and muscle tension, that occur in response to a perceived threat.

gamma-aminobutyric acid (GABA): a neurotransmitter that helps decrease brain activity. Some medications produce a calming effect through their influence on GABA.

generalized anxiety disorder (GAD): a psychiatric disorder characterized by a pattern of frequent, persistent worry and anxiety about several events or activities causing significant distress or impairment

institutional racism: patterns and policies that enforce discrimination based on race

neurotransmitters: chemicals in the brain that enable the transmission of electrical impulses between nerve cells, thus enabling communication between those nerve cells. They are vital to many physiological and psychological processes necessary for our survival.

norepinephrine: also called noradrenaline, a hormone and neurotransmitter produced by the adrenal glands and also secreted from nerve endings. A precursor to adrenaline, it works with adrenaline to cause an increase in heart rate, blood pressure, mental activity, blood flow to the muscles, and metabolism. This prepares a person to deal with stress or perceived threats.

obsessions: persistent, unwanted, irrational impulses, ideas, images, or thoughts that intrude into a person's consciousness, often causing intense anxiety and distress

obsessive-compulsive disorder (OCD): a neurobehavioral disorder in which people have obsessions, compulsions, or both that are time-consuming, distressing, or disruptive to usual routines, relationships with others, or daily functioning

panic attack: a frightening experience of brief but very intense fear that occurs "out of the blue" and is accompanied by physical symptoms, such as elevated heart rate, shortness of breath, dizziness, sweating, and nausea

panic disorder: a disorder in which a person has brief episodes (panic attacks) of intense fear accompanied by physical symptoms, such as elevated heart rate, shortness of breath, dizziness, sweating, and nausea. The person also has an ongoing preoccupation with the fear of having another panic attack.

post-traumatic stress disorder (PTSD): a psychiatric disorder characterized by highly distressing psychological and physical symptoms following exposure to a traumatic event involving extreme danger to oneself or others

predisposition: something that makes a person susceptible to a condition

psychotherapy: treatment for a mental or emotional disorder by analyzing behaviors and thoughts, especially through verbal communication with a medical professional

relaxation response: a state of deep relaxation with reduced heart rate, respiration, blood pressure, and muscle tension brought on by specific techniques of self-regulation, such as deep breathing, hypnosis, yoga, meditation, or progressive muscle relaxation

selective serotonin reuptake inhibitors (SSRIs): a group of antidepressants that work by increasing the amount of serotonin available to the nerve cells in the brain

serotonin: a neurotransmitter that is vital to the brain's capacity to properly regulate moods and control hunger, sleep, and aggression. An imbalance of serotonin contributes to anxiety and major mood disorders.

social phobia: also called social anxiety disorder, a psychiatric disorder characterized by severe anxiety in social situations. People with social phobia fear that the scrutiny of others will result in their being horribly embarrassed or humiliated or that others will think badly of them.

specific phobia: a psychiatric disorder involving an excessive or unreasonable fear of one particular type of object or situation

stage fright: a phrase to describe social phobia that is associated with artistic-performing fears

stress: a state of mental, emotional, or physical strain or tension or a combination of these from very demanding circumstances or psychological pressures

stress management: the active practice of a set of methods and techniques that promote effective coping with the stressors of daily living and combat stress-related diseases, such as high blood pressure, diabetes, or heart disease

SOURCE NOTES

5   Emma Pattee, "The Difference between Worry, Stress, and Anxiety," *New York Times*, February 26, 2020, https://www.nytimes.com/2020/02/26 /smarter-living/the-difference-between-worry-stress-and-anxiety.html.

11   Jessica DuLong, "Grief-Induced Anxiety: Calming the Fears That Follow Loss," CNN, July 18, 2021, https://www.cnn.com/2021/07/18/health /grief-anxiety-healing-loss-wellness/index.html.

27   Matt Richtel, "Surgeon General Warns of Youth Mental Health Crisis," *New York Times*, December 7, 2021, https://www.nytimes.com/2021/12/07 /science/pandemic-adolescents-depression-anxiety.html.

88   Selena Gomez (@selenagomez), "a note from me," Instagram photo, April 29, 2021, https://www.instagram.com/p/COQhmZrjITq/.

88   Megan McCluskey, "John Green on Mental Illness and Writing a Book That Mirrors His Own Life," *Time*, October 12, 2017, https://time.com /4976944/john-green-turtles-all-the-way-down-mental-illness/.

89   Brittney McNamara, "Ariana Grande Is Giving Away $2 Million in Free Therapy with BetterHelp," *Teen Vogue*, June 30, 2021, https://www .teenvogue.com/story/ariana-grande-is-giving-away-dollar1-million-in -free-therapy-with-betterhelp.

SELECTED BIBLIOGRAPHY

American Psychiatric Association. *Diagnostic and Statistical Manual of Mental Disorders*. 5th ed. Washington, DC: American Psychiatric Association, 2013.

Antony, Martin M., and Richard P. Swinson. *The Shyness and Social Anxiety Workbook: Proven Techniques for Overcoming Your Fears*. Oakland: New Harbinger, 2000.

Barlow, D. H. *Anxiety and Its Disorders*. New York: Guilford, 2002.

Bourne, Edmund. *The Anxiety and Phobia Workbook*. 3rd ed. Oakland: New Harbinger, 2000.

Davidson, Jonathan, and Henry Dreher. *The Anxiety Book: Developing Strength in the Face of Fear*. New York: Riverhead Books, 2003.

"Facts & Statistics." Anxiety and Depression Association of America. Accessed February 22, 2022.
https://adaa.org/about-adaa/press-room/facts-statistics.

Himle, Joseph A., Raymond E. Baser, Robert Joseph Taylor, Rosalyn Denise Campbell, and James S. Jackson. "Anxiety Disorders among African Americans, Blacks of Caribbean Descent, and Non-Hispanic Whites in the United States." *Journal of Anxiety Disorders* 23, no. 5 (June 2009): 578–590.
https://www.ncbi.nlm.nih.gov/pmc/articles/PMC4187248/.

Hyman, Bruce M., and Cherry Pedrick. *Obsessive-Compulsive Disorder*. Minneapolis: Twenty-First Century Books, 2011.

———. *The OCD Workbook: Your Guide to Breaking Free from Obsessive-Compulsive Disorder*. 3rd ed. Oakland: New Harbinger, 2010.

"Mental Health by the Numbers." National Alliance on Mental Illness. Last modified March 2021
https://www.nami.org/learn-more/mental-health-by-the-numbers.

"Any Anxiety Disorder." National Institute of Mental Health. Accessed February 22, 2022.
https://www.nimh.nih.gov/health/statistics/any-anxiety-disorder.shtml.

RESOURCES

These organizations can provide further information about anxiety disorders. They may be able to provide the names of local doctors and therapists who treat anxiety disorders. They don't always track the treatment practices of the professionals. So being on a list does not necessarily mean that a professional is competent to treat anxiety disorders. It only means that they have indicated an expertise or interest in treating one or more anxiety disorders.

Anxiety and Depression Association of America
8701 Georgia Ave., Ste. 412
Silver Spring, MD 20910
https://www.adaa.org

Association for Behavioral and Cognitive Therapies
305 Seventh Ave., 16th Fl.
New York, NY 10001-6008
https://www.abct.org

International Foundation for Research and Education on Depression (iFred)
PO Box 17598
Baltimore, MD 21297-1598
https://www.ifred.org/

International OCD Foundation
PO Box 961029
Boston, MA 02196
https://iocdf.org/

Obsessive Compulsive Information Center
Madison Institute of Medicine
6515 Grand Teton Plaza, Ste. 100
Madison, WI 53719
https://www.miminc.org

OCD Action
Suite 506–507, Davina House, 137–149
Goswell Rd., London EC1V 7ET
https://ocdaction.org.uk

FURTHER READING

Books for Young Adults

Earl, Rae. *Your Brain Needs a Hug: Life, Love, Mental Health, and Sandwiches.* New York: Imprint, 2019.

Galanti, Regine. *Anxiety Relief for Teens: Essential CBT Skills and Mindfulness Practices to Overcome Anxiety and Stress.* New York: Zeitgeist, 2020.

Hershfield, Jon. *The OCD Workbook for Teens: Mindfulness and CBT Skills to Help You Overcome Unwanted Thoughts and Compulsions.* Oakland: New Harbinger, 2021.

Kissen, Debra. *Rewire Your Anxious Brain for Teens: Using CBT, Neuroscience, and Mindfulness to Help You End Anxiety, Panic, and Worry.* Oakland: New Harbinger, 2020.

Sonenklar, Carol, and Tabitha Moriarty. *Not Just about Food: Understanding Eating Disorders.* Minneapolis: Twenty-First Century Books, 2023.

Sperling, Jacqueline. *Find Your Fierce: How to Put Social Anxiety in Its Place.* Washington, DC: Magination, 2021.

Tompkins, Michael A. *Zero to 60: A Teen's Guide to Manage Frustration, Anger, and Everyday Irritations.* Washington, DC: Magination, 2020.

Toner, Jacqueline B., and Claire A. B. Freeland. *Depression: A Teen's Guide to Survive and Thrive.* Washington, DC: Magination, 2016.

Wells, Polly. *Freaking Out: Real-Life Stories about Anxiety.* Toronto: Annick, 2013.

For Parents and Family Members

Browne, Jennifer, and Cody Buchanan. *Understanding Teenage Anxiety: A Parent's Guide to Improving Your Teen's Mental Health.* New York: Skyhorse, 2019.

Damour, Lisa. *Under Pressure: Confronting the Epidemic of Stress and Anxiety in Girls.* New York: Ballantine Books, 2019.

Duffy, John. *Parenting the New Teen in the Age of Anxiety: A Complete Guide to Your Child's Stressed, Depressed, Expanded, Amazing Adolescence.* Coral Gables, FL: Mango, 2019.

Zucker, Bonnie. *Parenting Kids with OCD: A Guide to Understanding and Supporting Your Child with OCD*. Waco, TX: Prufrock, 2017.

Websites

Center for Psychiatric Rehabilitation
> https://cpr.bu.edu/
> This is a website for people with a psychiatric condition that addresses issues and reasonable accommodations related to work and school, including information about the Americans with Disabilities Act (ADA), links to other school- and work-related sites, and advice for coping at school and work.

Internet Mental Health
> https://mentalhealth.com/home/
> Find more information about anxiety disorders and mental illness.

National Alliance on Mental Illness (NAMI)
> http://www.nami.org/Home
> NAMI is a national organization with affiliates in every state and more than eleven hundred communities with the mission of support, education, advocacy, and research for people living with mental illness. The website has information on OCD and other disorders, including interactive bulletin boards and links to state NAMI affiliates. Also included are Child and Teen Support, Veterans Resources, Multicultural Action Center, and FaithNet.

National Institute of Mental Health (NIMH)
> http://www.nimh.nih.gov
> The NIMH is part of the US Department of Health and Human Services. The NIMH's mission is to reduce the burden of mental illness and behavioral disorders through research on mind, brain, and behavior. The website provides access to professional journals and the latest research and statistics.

National Suicide Prevention Lifeline
> https://suicidepreventionlifeline.org
> 800-273-8255
> This site has information about suicide and a search tool for finding a crisis center near you. There is also a toll-free, twenty-four-hour hotline for those in crisis or thinking about suicide.

Psychology Today: Find a Therapist
https://www.psychologytoday.com/us/therapists
This site helps connect patients with therapists in the United States. The website allows users to filter potential therapists by location, specialty, health insurance coverage, and more.

INDEX

ABOUT THE AUTHORS

Cherry Pedrick, RN, is a retired registered nurse and a freelance writer living in Lacey, Washington. With Bruce Hyman, she is the coauthor of *The OCD Workbook: Your Guide to Breaking Free from Obsessive-Compulsive Disorder*, 3rd edition, and *Obsessive-Compulsive Disorder*. Pedrick is also the coauthor of *The Habit Change Workbook: How to Break Bad Habits and Form New Ones*, *The BDD Workbook: Overcome Body Dysmorphic Disorder and Body Image Obsessions*, *Helping Your Child with OCD*, and *Loving Someone with OCD*.

Bruce M. Hyman, PhD, LCSW, was in private practice in Hollywood/Fort Lauderdale, Florida, and was the director of the OCD Resource Center of Florida. He is the coauthor of *The OCD Workbook: Your Guide to Breaking Free from Obsessive-Compulsive Disorder*, 3rd edition; *Obsessive-Compulsive Disorder*; and *Coping with OCD: Practical Strategies for Living Well with OCD*. He specialized in the cognitive behavioral treatment of adults and children with OCD and other anxiety disorders.

Tabitha Moriarty is a medical student living in Atlanta, Georgia.

PHOTO ACKNOWLEDGMENTS

Image credits: LKW/Independent Picture Service, pp. 8, 21, 36; KM/ Independent Picture Service, p. 12; H.S. Photos/Alamy Stock Photo, p. 15; Boy_Anupong/Getty Images, p. 17; Sanna Lindberg/Getty Images, p. 19; DeymosHR/Shutterstock.com, p. 24; SEBASTIAN KAULITZKI/SCIENCE PHOTO LIBRARY/Getty Images, p. 25; Nopparat Khokthong/Shutterstock.com, p. 27; Monkey Business Images/Shutterstock.com, p. 29; MaFelipe/Getty Images, p. 32; Moyo Studio/Getty Images, p. 34; Central Press/Getty Images, p. 38; KatarzynaBialasiewicz/Getty Images, p. 48; Dougal Waters/Getty Images, p. 54; goc/Getty Images, p. 57; BSIP/Education Images/Universal Images Group/Getty Images, p. 59; Blamb/Shutterstock.com, p. 61; fizkes/ Shutterstock.com, p. 63; SolStock/Getty Images, p. 69; Jasmina007/Getty Images, p. 73; Peter Griffith/Getty Images, p. 75; Jonathan Schneider/EyeEm/ Getty Images, p. 76; Thomas Barwick/Getty Images, p. 78; Peter Snaterse/ Shutterstock.com, p. 81; Sladic/Getty Images, p. 86; Tibrina Hobson/Getty Images, p. 89. Design elements: VectorPlotnikoff/Shutterstock.com; Rashad Ashur/Shutterstock.com; viktorov.pro/Shutterstock.com.
Cover image: ZaZa Studio/Shutterstock.com.